OVERCOMING OPPOSITIONAL DEFIANT DISORDER & ATTENTION DEFICIT HYPERACTIVITY DISORDER:

A parent's guide To Better Understand and Manage ODD and ADHD in Their Children

By Cathryn Guglielminetti

OPPOSITIONAL DEFIANT DISORDER

HOW TO MANAGE AND OVERCOME ODD

By

Cathryn Guglielminetti

TABLE OF CONTENTS

INTRODUCTION

While most children will periodically be opposite, especially when weary or stressed out, children with Oppositional Defiant Disorder (ODD) have a continuous pattern of disobedience and hostility towards parents, instructors, and other authorities as well as refuse to follow grownups' requests. They are additionally usually quickly irritated and regularly lose their temper. ODD and various other conduct troubles are the best reasons for referral to children's mental health services.

There are numerous people all throughout the United States that have actually had the bad luck of coming down with some kind of behavioral condition. Frequently, these conditions are intensified due to the reality that the child is not fully mature to understand what is really taking place to them, nor do they have the vocabulary to discuss what they are feeling, so, rather, they snap a lot more at their siblings and the grownups in their lives. One such syndrome that this often occurs with is Oppositional Defiant Disorder, or ODD for brief. As the name recommends, children who experience ODD are usually openly and angrily defiant of those in their lives - particularly adults that seek to suppress their actions with regulations or requests which they consider as an invasion. This brings about considerably defiant, sometimes ruthless habits in the child as well as which leaves parents unsure of how to manage them. It is consequently that many parents often neglect their daring child, leading them to really worsen, creating even more problems as well as possibly developing the foundation for a lot more noticeable behavior problems later on in life.

Little children have outbursts, and bigger children can be irritable, snotty and moody. So, just how do you know when it's a challenging stage or when there is a bigger issue developing that needs interest? A child need not rise to the degree of harming pets or people, damaging property or stealing, to have a diagnosable issue that requires therapy.

Oppositional Defiant Disorder is a repeated pattern of emoting and acting out that lasts for at least six (6) months, and also is especially guided towards some authority figure in their lives, such as an instructor, parent, or teacher. It is another problem called conduct disorder, if the aggression is physical.

Do you have children that have Oppositional Defiant Disorder (ODD)? Are you having problem dealing with ODD? Parenting is challenging due to the fact that other than offering them all the physical resources they require, parents require to provide care, love, and attention. If you are a mom and/or dad whose child has behavior problems like Oppositional Defiant Disorder (ODD), for sure, you feel worn out, angry, annoyed or perhaps disappointed.

It would actually be abnormal if a child was not defiant every now and then. When this behavior becomes the normal everyday behavior, your child may have ODD.

If left untreated, this condition can lead not only to more problems at home but major problems when the child gets into school. Your ODD child can drive you absolutely nuts at times. As parents it's up to us to ensure they get treated and have a fair shot at life.

Among the symptoms of an ODD child is they intend to suggest regarding everything they are asked to do. They may intentionally try to make other individuals upset, annoyed, or unhappy. They argue with grownups about every little thing. They constantly tease or try to aggravate their brother or sisters.

As you can visualize, this actions can trigger major issues in institution as the child will disrespect authority as well as usually end up in conflicts. In addition, as the child grows older, these "small" defiance issues might develop into legal trouble or several other serious problems.

If you are among these parents, it is important for you to understand what ODD is, its features and methods of managing the disorder correctly. Care and love is not nearly enough due to the fact that ODD is not an ordinary disorder that can be addressed by plain understanding as well as dedication, but you need to get in touch with child behavior expert to understand the most effective treatment available.

WHAT IS ODD?

The causes of ODD are not yet acknowledged but there are two (2) important hypotheses which describe the advancement of Oppositional Defiant Disorder in a child. Developmental professionals imply that ODD begins throughout a childhood.

A child who endures Oppositional Defiant Disorder has a greater challenge in learning because their focus is distracted by the defiance of authority particularly in institution, which hinders obtaining skills to do things independently. Another theory of the reasons for ODD is the suppressed corrective approaches made use of by experts and parents alike. Using unresponsive disciplinary actions reinforces opposite habits in a child. Parents ought to undertake parent management training which concentrates on teaching parents of children with ODD more efficient, certain techniques for taking care of the child's opposition as well as defiance.

The majority of individuals with ODD including teenagers, which consists of 23% of school-aged children. Symptoms of children with the problem are seen as very early as the age of 2 or 3 years old, and throughout the pubescent years. Children with

ODD have the same actions even if they are not tired, starving or stressed out, which gets in the means of discovering and also a child's ability to form partnerships with others.

Oppositional Defiant Disorder in children indicates the frequent pattern of disobedient, hostile, and defiant behavior towards parents, elders or elderly authorities like educators. Bold behavior is considered typical amongst the children of two to 3 years of age as well as among early adolescents. If the habits of a child is found to be different from other children and it is lingering for years, after that he has actually certainly developed ODD.

ODD intensifies the already disorderly and also difficult homelife of a child. Such defiant children are the victims of their very own proneness, which disable them to go against the defined laws. These children really feel enjoyment in purposely vexing other individuals.

The occurrence of ODD is somewhere related to the kind of structure existing at the home of a child. Apart from this factor, ODD is also linked with one more adolescent behavioral disorder, i.e., Reactive Attachment Disorder, whereby a child is not supported with the sufficient treatment as well as interest during his early stage. Throughout the course of his development, this attachment problem additionally grows as well as he may acquire the undesirable characteristics of bold children.

Children with the problem often hold other people responsible for their activities as well as will probably enter discussions very quickly. They have stress and anxiety concerns, use discourteous language, detect the awful high qualities of others as well as are deliberately very rude. These are some signs of children with ODD, also when you notice these signs &symptoms in your very own children,

In addition, the best-behaved children can be difficult and also tough at times. If your child or teenager has a consistent as well as constant pattern of rage, irritability, shouting, defiance, or vindictiveness towards you and other authority figures, he or she might have ODD.

As parents, you do not have to go it alone in trying to manage a child with ODD. Doctors, mental health professionals as well as child development experts can help.

Behavior treatment of ODD includes discovering skills to assist in building positive home interactions as well as to take care of problematic actions. Added therapy, and perhaps medicines, might be required to treat related mental health problems.

DOES YOUR CHILD'S BEHAVIOR SHOW SIGNS OF OPPOSITIONAL DEFIANT DISORDER?

Sometimes it's difficult to acknowledge the distinction in between an emotional or strong-willed child and one with Oppositional Defiant Disorder. It's typical to exhibit oppositional behavior at specific phases of a child's growth.

Signs of ODD generally begin during preschool years. Often ODD might establish later, yet usually before the very early teenager years. These habits trigger substantial ill health at home, social tasks, school, and job.

The majority of signs and symptoms seen in children and also teenagers with ODD also occur sometimes in other children without it. This is extremely real for children around ages 2 or 3, or throughout the teen years. Numerous children often tend to disobey, argue with parents or resist authority. They might usually behave in this manner when they are exhausted, starving, or trouble. But in children as well as teenagers with

ODD, these signs and symptoms take place more often. They likewise hinder learning as well as educational development as well as sometimes, they interfere with the child's partnerships with others

The Diagnostic and Statistical Manual of Mental Disorders (DSM-5), released by the American Psychiatric Association, provides criteria for diagnosing ODD. The DSM-5 requirements consist of behavior and emotional signs and symptoms that last at least six months. These include:

Angry and also short-tempered mood:

- Typically and conveniently loses temper
- Is often sensitive as well as easily annoyed by others
- Is resentful and also frequently mad

Defiant and argumentative habits:

- Commonly argues with grownups or individuals in authority
- Often proactively declines or opposes to comply with adults' requests or regulations
- Frequently deliberately frustrates or upsets people
- Usually blames others for his or her errors or misbehavior

Spite:

- Is vindictive or usually spiteful
- Has actually revealed hurtful or spiteful actions at least two times in the past 6 months

Others signs:

- Tossing repeated temper tantrums
- Excessively arguing with adults, particularly those with authority
- Actively rejecting to adhere to policies as well as requests
- Intentionally trying to frustrate or disturb others, or being conveniently annoyed by others
- Criticizing others for your errors
- Having frequent outbursts of anger and also animosity
- Being spiteful as well as seeking retribution
- Swearing or utilizing profane language
- Saying mean as well as hateful things when distressed

Additionally, many children with ODD are moody, quickly disappointed as well as have a reduced self-esteem. They likewise often might abuse alcohol and drugs.

ODD can differ in intensity:

- Light: Symptoms occur just in one setting, such as just in the house, college, work or with peers.
- Modest: Some signs and symptoms occur in at least two (2) setups.
- Serious: Some signs take place in three or more setups.
- For some children, symptoms may initially be seen only in the house, but with time extend to various other setups, such as college and with good friends.

WHAT CAUSES ODD?

The exact root cause of ODD is unidentified, though many experts map it back to a combination of mental, social, and also natural elements. ODD signs are commonly connected to prenatal smoke exposure, contaminant direct exposure, or inadequate nutrition. ODD is much more common in individuals that have loved ones with ODD, ADHD, Conduct Disorder (CD), mood problems, or substance abuse problems. Though researchers have actually not pinpointed a specific gene responsible, traumatic life occasions, like childhood abuse, can activate ODD for some people.

To identify ODD accurately, a doctor will perform an assessment to rule out anxiousness or state of mind conditions, which can all trigger ODD-like behaviors. These habits are just "signs" of ODD if they occur more frequently than is regular for people of the same age and developing degree, as well as if they cause scientifically substantial impairment in social, scholastic, or work functioning.

An assessing physician might put together an in-depth actions background from parents, instructors, as well as professional monitoring. Talking to as many individuals as possible about how and also where the actions happens can assist the medical professional figure out which actions are influencing different areas of the child's life.

An individual with ODD hardly ever takes responsibility for her habits and also the effect it has on everyone around them. She sees "the trouble" lying with any person but herself. It typically takes a highly certified doctor to establish whether problems at job, institution, or residence trace back to ODD.

Before detecting oppositional defiant disorder, the medical professional needs to rule out problems such as a mood condition (particularly bipolar range disorder), personality disorders (particularly borderline, narcissistic as well as antisocial personality disorders), injury (physical or sexual assault), as well as drug abuse. Each of these can trigger oppositional actions and ODD signs and symptoms.

The pressure of handling ODD affects the entire family members, and also might strain marriage partnerships. The good news is, effective treatments exist for controlling also one of the most out of control child or grownup. Altering behaviors is not easy, however, it can be done – normally with the help of specialized psychotherapy, a medical professional to manage treatment, and sometimes medication.

The exact reason for ODD is not known, yet it is believed that a mix of organic, genetic, and environmental elements might add to the condition.

Biological: Some studies recommend that problems in or injuries to particular locations of the mind can lead to serious behavioral problems in children. Furthermore, ODD has actually been linked to abnormal functioning of particular sorts of mind chemicals, or neurotransmitters. Neurotransmitters assist nerve cells in the mind interact with each other. If these chemicals are not functioning appropriately, messages might deficient via the brain correctly, leading to signs of ODD, and also other mental illnesses. Even more, numerous children and teens with ODD also have other mental illnesses, such as ADHD, discovering disorders, anxiety, or a stress and anxiety disorder, which may contribute to their troubling actions.

Genes: Many children as well as teenagers with ODD have close family members with mental illnesses, consisting of mood conditions, stress and anxiety disorders, and also personality disorders. This suggests that a susceptibility to establish ODD may be acquired.

Environmental: Factors such as an ineffective family life, a family history of mental illnesses and/or chemical abuse, and also inconsistent discipline by parents might contribute to the development of habits conditions.

Scientists do not understand what creates ODD. There are two (2) major theories for why it occurs:

Developing theory: When children are toddlers, this concept suggests that the problems begin. Children and teens with ODD might have had difficulty learning to become independent from a parent or various other primary person to whom they were emotionally attached. Their behavior may be typical developing issues that are lasting past the toddler years.

Understanding theory: This theory suggests that the negative symptoms of ODD are found out perspectives. They mirror the effects of unfavorable reinforcement methods used by parents as well as others in power. Using negative reinforcement increases the child's ODD actions. That's due to the fact that these actions permit the child to obtain what he or she wants: interest and also reaction from others or parents.

Risk factors

Oppositional defiant disorder is a complex problem. Possible danger variables for ODD include:

Temperament – a child who has a character that includes difficulty controlling feelings, such as being very emotionally responsive to circumstances or having trouble enduring stress.

Parenting issues – a child who experiences abuse or disregard, inconsistent or difficult self-control, or an absence of adult supervision.

Other home problems –a child that lives with parent or home discord or has a parent with a mental health and wellness or substance utilize disorder.

Atmosphere – oppositional and also bold actions can be reinforced and also enhanced via focus from peers as well as inconsistent self-control from other authority numbers, such as teachers.

Complications

Children and also teens with ODD may have trouble at home with parents and also siblings, in college with teachers, and at the workplace with supervisors and various other authority figures. Children with ODD might have a hard time to make and maintain partnerships and also good friends.

ODD might result in problems such as:

- Poor college and also work performance

- Antisocial behavior

- Impulse control problems

- Substance Abuse

- Suicide

Manychildren and also teenagers with ODD additionally have various other mental health and wellness problems, such as:

- Attention-deficit/hyperactivity condition (ADHD).

- Behavior problem

- Depression

- Anxiety

- Learning and communication problems

Dealing with these various other psychological health disorders may assist enhance ODD signs. If these various other conditions are not reviewed and also treated properly, it might be hard to deal with ODD.

WHAT IS THE DIFFERENCE BETWEEN COMMON DISOBEDIENCE AND ODD?

ODD and Conduct Disorder

How do you respond to an adolescent who gets up as well as obstructs your method when you're attempting to leave the room, towering over you and looking at you in a method that makes your tummy pains? Is this oppositional defiant disorder or perform disorder, and also just how can you deal with this?

We chat every day with parents who feel their dream of growing a child has actually transformed into a parenting problem. Our focus is on understanding and reacting to this actions, while supporting a certain team of parents that frequently feel isolated and also as if no one comprehends their circumstance.

Is it Oppositional Defiant Disorder (ODD) or Conduct Disorder?

Many parents and also specialists have trouble identifying the distinctions in between ODD and Conduct Disorder related actions. ODD is identified by a child or young adult that disputes with authority figures, such as instructors and also parents.

The defining feature is a struggle against being managed. For a child like this, being controlled feels like drowning. Conduct problem is made use of to explain an older child or adolescent who has actually moved into a pattern of violating the rights of others: scare tactics or aggression toward pets or individuals, swiping or the calculated devastation of property.

If a next-door neighbor's child was literally intimidating you, what would certainly you do? Stay clear of escalating the scenario.

A key difference in between ODD and Conduct Disorder exists in the role of control. Children that have actually started to move – or have currently moved – into conduct problem will combat not just against being managed, but will try to regulate others. If you think your teen is moving into conduct disorder – or if you recognize he's already there– right here are five (5) things that can assist you.

Parenting a Child with Conduct Disorder

Acknowledge the circumstance. No parent anticipates to be faced eventually with their own child's intimidation as well as perhaps prohibited actions. It can be tempting to excuse the behavior or rationalize, but that will only make things worse. Approving the fact of the circumstance doesn't indicate you are approving your teenager's habits. It implies you are acknowledging, "This is what it is, today, presently." It gives you a starting point for exactly how to react to the behavior.

If you're parenting a teenager who's involving in intimidation, aggression, or various other conduct disordered actions, those life areas become high-ends. If you're not able to deal with intimidating actions without showing worry, stay clear of the situation as a lot as possible. Again, this isn't accepting the behavior, it's accepting the fact.

Safety and security is tough to achieve if you have not acknowledged the situation for what it is. Prevention is a key concern when responding to Conduct Disorder behavior. Don't have family pets if your child is harsh to animals. Do not leave her alone with younger siblings if your little girl is aggressive. Do not go in there if your boy is aggressive with you if you go in his space. If your child comes to be violent when you ask about homework, do not ask. Here's the fact: if she does not do her homework, she will stop working. That occurs. If she's old enough to frighten you, she's old enough to understand that she needs to complete classwork in order to pass to the next grade.

Avoid blame. Placing blame for your child's behavior is a waste of time. Don't blame yourself, your child's other parent, friends/peers, or even your child. Definitely hold him responsible, however, blame will certainly leave you feeling resentful as well as mad. Your child is making choices that will have effects– potentially long-term consequences. He is responsible for those selections. Bear in mind, a strong feature of conduct disorder is controlling others. Getting you to take responsibility for adverse behavior is a kind of manipulation. Blaming yourself will leave you really feeling guilty and also keep you from reacting effectively to these habits as a parent

You might choose to stay clear of particular situations in order to decrease the potential for escalation, that doesn't suggest you need to hand over control of your very own habits and also choices to your child. Do not compensate habits that breaches the rights of others. This might sound rough, yet this is significant behavior, and while you don't want to increase it, you also don't want to reinforce it.

Get help. Discover a therapist that comprehends Conduct Disorder. Go yourself if your child declines to participate in treatment. Handling Conduct Disorder is among the hardest obstacles parents can face. Do not attempt to do it alone. You require assistance.

As parents and also therapists, we understand this was a tough post to check out if you're facing this type of habits with your child. The information we supply below is genuinely just a little slice of parenting a teenager who is involving in intimidation, aggressiveness or various other serious behavior.

ODD vs. ADHD

The Facts About Oppositional Defiant Disorder as well as Attention Deficit

About 40 percent (40%) of children with attention deficit disorder (ADHD or ADD) likewise have Oppositional Defiant Disorder (ODD) or a related conduct problem. Could your child's disobedience, defiance, as well as rage be symptoms of ODD? Figure out everything you need to learn about the ADHD versus ODD link.

Oppositional defiant disorder (ODD) is defined by aggression and a propensity to purposefully trouble and also irritate others. While it holds true that anybody can be hostile and also annoying once in a while, to be identified as ODD, an individual should display a pattern of negativistic, hostile, as well as defiant actions lasting at least six months.

Some sources approximate that five percent (5%) of all children may get the medical diagnosis.

What's the Difference Between ADHD and also ODD?

Not all children with attention deficit disorder (ADHD or ADD) receive the ODD medical diagnosis. Nevertheless, the portions are high– some researches put price quotes as high as 65 percent of children with ADHD that additionally have a defiance condition. A recent article in *Attention!*, the quarterly magazine released by CHADD, mentions a research of 600 childrento 9 years of age in which 40 percent of the children with ADHD also had ODD, with 15 percent, or 1 in 7, having a lot more severe conduct problems.

What is ADHD?

Attention Deficit Hyperactivity Disorder (ADHD) is a mental health and wellness problem that can cause above-normal levels of hyperactive and also impulsive habits. People with ADHD might likewise have difficulty focusing their attention on a solitary job or sitting still for long periods of time.

Both children and adults can have ADHD. It's a medical diagnosis the American Psychiatric Association (APA) recognizes.

ADHD signs

A large range of behaviors are connected with ADHD. Some of the more typical ones consist of:

- having difficulty concentrating or focusing on tasks

- being forgetful regarding completing jobs

- being easily distracted

- having trouble sitting still

- interrupting people while they're chatting

You may have some or all of these symptoms if you or your child has ADHD. The signs and symptoms you have, rely on the type of ADHD you have

Typical indications of ADHD in children:

1. Self-focused actions

A usual sign of ADHD is what appears like an inability to identify other individuals' requirements and desires. This can cause the next two indicators: disrupting as well as trouble waiting their turn.

2. Disrupting

Self-focused actions may create a child with ADHD to disturb others while they're chatting or butt into video games or discussions they're not part of.

3. Problem waiting their turn

Children with ADHD may have problem waiting their turn during class activities or when playing video games with other children.

4. Psychological turmoil

A child with ADHD may have problem maintaining their emotions in check. They may have outbursts of rage at unsuitable times. Youngerchildren may have tantrums.

5. Fidgetiness

Children with ADHD often can't sit still. They might attempt to stand up and run around, fidget, or wriggle in their chair when required to rest.

6. Problems playing silently

Fidgetiness can make it challenging for children with ADHD to play quietly or engage steadily in pastime.

7. Incomplete jobs

A child with ADHD might show interest in great deals of different goals, however, they might have problems finishing them. They may start tasks, tasks, or homework, but move on to the following thing that catches their rate of interest before completing.

8. Absence of emphasis

A child with ADHD may have trouble focusing, also when someone is talking straight to them. They'll say they heard you, yet they will not have the ability to repeat back to you what you just stated.

9. Evasion of jobs needing extensive psychological effort

This same absence of emphasis can trigger a child to stay clear of tasks that require a continual mental initiative, such as listening in class or doing research.

10. Mistakes

Children with ADHD can have trouble complying with guidelines that need planning or implementing a plan. This can then cause careless blunders– yet it doesn't show idleness or an absence of knowledge.

11. Imagining

Children with ADHD aren't loud and constantly rambunctious. Another indication of ADHD is being quieter as well as less engaged than various other children. A child with ADHD may stare right into room, musing, and overlook what's going on around them.

12. Trouble getting organized

A child with ADHD might have trouble monitoring tasks and activities. This might trigger problems at institution, as they can discover it tough to focus on research, institution jobs, as well as other tasks.

13. Lapse of memory

Children with ADHD might be absent-minded in everyday tasks. They may neglect to do jobs or their homework. They might likewise lose things frequently, such as toys.

14. Symptoms in several areas

A child with ADHD will show signs of the problem in greater than one setup. For example, they may show lack of focus both in institution and also in your home.

All children are most likely to display some of these habits eventually. Imagining, fidgeting, as well as consistent interruptions are all usual actions in children. You need to begin assuming about the following steps if:

- Your child regularly presents signs of ADHD
- This behavior is impacting their success in society and leading to negative communications with their peers

ADHD is treatable. Review all of the therapy choices if your child is diagnosed with ADHD. Then, establish a time to meet with a physician or psychotherapist to determine the very best course of action.

Types of ADHD

To make ADHD detects much more consistent, the APA has organized the problem into three categories, or types. These kinds are mainly primarily inattentive, primarily hyperactivity-impulsive, and a mix of both.

Primarily inattentive

As the name recommends, people with this kind of ADHD have extreme difficulty focusing, completing tasks, and also following directions.

Professionals also believe that numerous children with the inattentive kind of ADHD may not receive an appropriate medical diagnosis because they don't have a tendency to disrupt the classroom. This type is most typical among girls with ADHD.

Primarily hyperactive-impulsive

People with this type of ADHD show mostly hyper and spontaneous behavior. This can include fidgeting, interrupting individuals while they're speaking, and also not having the ability to wait their turn.

Negligence is much less of a worry with this type of ADHD. Individuals with mainly hyperactive-impulsive ADHD may still find it difficult to focus on tasks.

Integrated Primarily Inattentive as well as Primarily Hyperactive-impulsive type

This is the most usual sort of ADHD. Individuals with this combined kind of ADHD display both apathetic and also hyperactive signs. These consist of a failure to take note, a propensity toward spontaneity, and also above-normal levels of activity and energy.

The kind of ADHD you or your child has will determine how it's dealt with. The type you have can transform in time, so your treatment may alter, as well. Discover more concerning the three types of ADHD.

Adult ADHD.

Greater than 60 percent of children with ADHD still exhibit signs and symptoms as grownups. However, for many people, ADHD signs reduce or end up being much less constant as they get older.

That said, treatment is necessary. Without treatment, ADHD in grownups can have an unfavorable impact on numerous facets of life. Symptoms such as difficulty handling time, lapse of memory as well as rashness, can cause problems at work, home as well as in all kinds of partnerships. Figure out more regarding the signs and symptoms of ADHD in adults and how they can affect your life.

ADHD in children

One in 10 children between ages 5 to 17 years receives an ADHD medical diagnosis, making this set of one of the most common childhood neuro developmental problems in the United States.

For children, ADHD is normally connected with issues at school. Children with ADHD typically have trouble doing well in a controlled class setting.

Young boys are greater than twice as likely as girls to receive an ADHD diagnosis. This might be since boys tend to show characteristic symptoms of hyperactivity. Although some ladies with ADHD might have the timeless signs of hyperactivity, many do not. In most cases, women with ADHD might:

- daydream frequently

- be hyper-talkative as opposed to hyper

Many signs and symptoms of ADHD can be common childhood years actions, so it can be tough to know what's ADHD-related and also what's not.

What causes ADHD?

In spite of how usual ADHD is, researchers and physicians still aren't certain what triggers the problem. It's believed to have neurological beginnings. Genetics might likewise play a role.

Research suggests that a reduction in dopamine is a link toADHD. Dopamine is a chemical in the brain that helps move signals from one nerve to another. It contributes in setting off psychological reactions as well as motions.

Various other study recommends a structural difference in the mind. Findings show that individuals with ADHD have less gray matter quantity. Brainconsists of the mind areas that assist with:

- speech

- self-discipline

- decision-making

- muscle control

Researchers are still examining possible reasons for ADHD, such as smoking cigarettes while pregnant.

ADHD testing and also medical diagnosis

There's no single examination that can tell if you or your child has ADHD. A recent study highlighted the benefits of a brand-new test to diagnose adult

ADHD, yet numerous medical professionals think an ADHD medical diagnosis can't be made based upon one examination.

To make a diagnosis, your doctor will assess any type of symptoms you or your child has actually had over the previous six (6) months.

Your medical professional will likely gather info from instructors or relative as well as might use lists and also ranking scales to evaluate symptoms. They'll also do a physical examination to check for other illness.

Talk to your doctor about obtaining an examination if you suspect that you or your child has ADHD. For your child, you can also speak with their school counselor. Schools consistently examine children for troubles that might be impacting their instructional efficiency.

For the assessment, offer your physician or therapist with notes related to monitoring yourself or your child's habits.

They might refer you or your child to an ADHD expert if they suspect ADHD. Relying on the medical diagnosis, they may also suggest making a visit with a psychoanalyst or neurologist.

ADHD treatment

Therapy for ADHD commonly consists of behavioral therapies, medication, or both.

Types of therapy consist of psychiatric therapy, or talk therapy. With talk treatment, you or your child will certainly review exactly how ADHD affects your life and ways to help you handle it.

Another treatment type is behavioral therapy. This therapy can aid you or your child with discovering how to check and also handle your habits.

When you're living with ADHD, medicine can additionally be really handy. ADHD medicines are made to impact brain chemicals in such a way that enables you to far better control your activities and impulses.

ODD SYMPTOMS AND PREVALENCE

What are the signs of a defiance condition like ODD?

A pattern of negativistic, hostile, and defiant habits lasting at least six months, during which four (or even more) of the adhering to ODD signs and symptoms are present:

- often loses temper

- commonly argues with grownups

- often proactively resists or declines to comply with adults' requests or rules

- usually deliberately irritates people

- commonly condemns others for his/her mistakes or misdeed

- is typically sensitive or conveniently frustrated by others

- is resentful as well as frequently mad

- is ruthless or usually spiteful

Keep in mind: Consider a standard for ODD satisfied only if the actions takes place extra frequently than is commonly observed in people of similar age as well as in a developing degree.

A medical diagnosis of ODD is taken into consideration just if:

- The ODD behavior disruption creates clinically substantial problems in social, academic, or job-related functioning.
- The bold behaviors do not happen specifically during the program of a

psychotic episode or because of a state of mind disorder.

- Criteria are not satisfied for Conduct Disorder, and, if the individual is age 18 years or older, criteria are not met for Antisocial Personality Disorder. Find out more about Oppositional Defiant Disorder in grownups here.

Criteria summed up from American Psychiatric Association. Diagnostic and Statistical Manual of Mental Disorders, 5th version. Washington, DC: American Psychiatric Association.

Criteria to diagnose oppositional defiant disorder

A skilled psychiatrist or psychologist can identify children and also grownups with ODD. The Diagnostic as well as Statistical Manual of Mental Disorders, called the DSM-5, describes three (3) primary variables required to make a diagnosis of ODD:

1. They reveal a behavior pattern

An individual has to have a pattern of angry or short-tempered moods, argumentative or defiant behaviors, or spite long lasting a minimum of six months. During this moment, they need to display at the very least four of the following behaviors from any type of category.

A minimum of one of these signs and symptoms must be presented with someone that is not a sibling. The categories and also symptoms include:

Angry or short-tempered mood, that includes signs like:

- commonly shedding their mood

- being sensitive

- being easily irritated

- often becoming resentful or mad

Defiant or argumentative behavior, that includes signs and symptoms like:

- having frequent debates with authority figures or grownups

- actively opposing requests from authority numbers

- refusing to abide by demands from authority numbers

- purposely annoying others

- criticizing others for wrongdoing

- vindictiveness

- acting spitefully at least two times in a six-month period

2. The habits interrupts their life.

If the disruption in habits is associated with distress in the person or their instant social circle, the 2nd thing an expert looks for is. The turbulent actions might negatively affect important locations like their social life, education and learning, or occupation.

3. It's not connected to substance abuse or mental wellness episodes.

For medical diagnosis, the behaviors can't take place solely throughout the training course of episodes that include:

- substance abuse

- clinical depression

- bipolar disorder

- psychosis

- difficulty

The DSM-5 additionally has a range of intensity. A diagnosis of ODD can be:

- Mild: Symptoms are confined to just one setting.

- Moderate: Some signs and symptoms will certainly be present in a minimum of two setups.

- Severe: Symptoms will certainly be present in 3 or more setups.

TREATMENT FOR OPPOSITIONAL DEFIANT DISORDER

Early treatment is important for people with ODD. Teenagers as well as grownups with neglected ODD have raised danger for clinical depression and also chemical abuse, according to the American Academy of Child & Adolescent Psychiatry.

Treatment options can include:

Cognitive behavior modification

A talk therapy concentrated on changing unfavorable thoughts, behaviors and emotional reactions related to psychological distress.

Cognitive behavioral therapy (CBT) is a short-term, ambitious psychotherapy treatment that takes a hands-on, useful method to problem-solving. Its objective is to change patterns of believing or actions that lag individuals' troubles, and so transform the means they feel. It is used to assist in dealing with a vast array of concerns in a person's life, from sleeping problems or connection issues, to alcohol and drug misuse, or anxiety as well as clinical depression. CBT works by altering individuals' attitudes and also their behavior by concentrating on the thoughts, images, ideas and also mindsets that are held (a person's cognitive processes) and also just how these procedures connect to the method an individual acts, as a way of handling psychological problems.

Cognitive behavior treatment can be assumed of as a combination of psychiatric therapy and behavior therapy. Behavioral treatment pays close attention to the relationship in between our issues, our habits and our ideas.

The History of Cognitive Behavioral Therapy

Cognitive behavior modification was created by a psychoanalyst, Aaron Beck, in the 1960s. He was performing psychoanalysis at the time and also observed that throughout his analytical sessions, his people had a tendency to have an internal discussion taking place in their minds– virtually as if they were speaking to themselves. But they would only report a fraction of this type of believing to him.

In a treatment session the customer may be assuming to herself: "He (the specialist) hasn't stated much today." These ideas could make the client feel possibly irritated or a little distressed.

Beck realized that the link between ideas and sensations was extremely crucial. He created the term automated ideas to define emotion-filled ideas that could turn up in the mind. Beck discovered that individuals weren't constantly fully familiar with such ideas, however, could learn to determine as well as report them. The thoughts were usually unfavorable and also neither practical nor sensible if an individual was really feeling distressed in some means. Beck located that determining these thoughts was the essential to the customer understanding as well as overcoming his or her difficulties.

It's currently known as Cognitive-behavioral Treatment (CBT) because the treatment utilizes behavioral methods. The balance between the cognitive and also the behavioral components varies amongst the various treatments of this type, but all come under the umbrella term cognitive behavior treatment.

The Importance of Negative Thoughts

CBT is based on a model or concept that it's not occasions themselves that upset us, but the meanings we provide. It can block us seeing things or doing points that do not fit– that disconfirm– what we believe is real if our thoughts are also negative. To put it simply, we continue to hang on to the same old ideas and also fall short to find out anything brand-new.

A clinically depressed lady may assume, "I can't encounter going into work today; I can't do it." As an outcome of having these thoughts – as well as of believing them– she might well ring in sick. Thinking, acting, and feeling like this might begin a downward spiral.

Where Do These Negative Thoughts Come From?

Beck suggested that these thinking patterns are established in childhood, and also become automated and reasonably repaired. A child who really did not obtain much open affection from their parents yet was applauded for college job, might come to think, "I have to do well all the time. If I don't, individuals will certainly reject me." Such a policy for living (called an inefficient presumption) may succeed for the individual a lot of the moment and help them to work hard.

If something takes place that's past their control and also they experience failure, after that the dysfunctional idea pattern might be triggered. The individual might then begin to have automatic thoughts like, "I've completely failed.

Cognitive-behavioral treatment acts to assist the individual recognize that this is what's going on. It helps him or her to step outside their automated ideas and also test them out. CBT would certainly motivate the clinically depressed lady mentioned earlier to take a look at real-life experiences to see what happens to her, or to others, in similar scenarios. After that, in the light of a more practical point of view, she may be able to take the possibility of testing out what other individuals assume, by revealing something of her troubles to friends.

Clearly, adverse things can and do occur. When we are in a disrupted state of mind, we may be basing our predictions and analyses on a biased sight of the scenario, making the problem that we deal with seem much even worse. CBT aids people to deal with these misinterpretations.

Sorts Of Cognitive Behavior Therapy

According to the British Association of Behavioral and Cognitive Psychotherapies, "Cognitive and also behavior psychiatric therapies are a series of therapies based upon principles as well as concepts originated from psychological designs of human feeling and also actions. They consist of a vast array of treatment methods for mental illness, along a continuum from organized specific psychiatric therapy to self-help product."

There are a variety of certain types of restorative strategies that include CBT that are routinely used by mental wellness experts. Instances of these consist of:

Sensible Emotive Behavior Therapy (REBT): This type of CBT is fixated determining and changing unreasonable ideas. The procedure of REBT includes identifying the underlying irrational ideas, proactively challenging these ideas, and also finally discovering to acknowledge as well as alter these assumed patterns.

It is a type of cognitive-behavioral therapy created by psychotherapist Albert Ellis. REBT is concentrated on aiding clients transform unreasonable beliefs.

Let's take a closer look at how REBT was developed and how it works.

As a young man, Ellis located himself yearning for companionship yet experienced a severe worry of speaking to ladies. Over time, Ellis found that his fear of talking to women had reduced considerably.

Ellis later described that this experience worked as a basis for developing his technique to treatment, integrating behavioral strategies with examining underlying thoughts and also feelings. He had actually trained as a medical psychologist. He kept in mind that while his patients were able to end up being mindful of their hidden troubles, their actions did not necessarily transform as an outcome.

By the 1950s, Ellis had actually started trying out various other sorts of psychiatric therapy and was greatly affected by psycho therapists and theorists consisting of Karen Horney as well as Alfred Adler as well as the work of behavior specialists. Ellis's goal was to develop what he considered as an action-oriented method to psychotherapy designed to generate outcomes by helping customers manage their actions, cognitions, and also feelings.

According to Ellis, "Individuals are not disturbed by things however rather by their view of points." The fundamental assertion of REBT is that the method people really feel is largely affected by just how they believe. When people hold illogical beliefs about themselves or the world, problems can result.

The objective of REBT is to help individuals modify to not logical ideas and adverse thinking patterns in order to get rid of emotional issues and psychological distress due to this.

REBT was among the extremely initial sorts of cognitive treatments. Ellis first started creating REBT throughout the very early 1950s and also initially called his approach to logical therapy. In 1959, the method was redubbed Reasonable Emotive Treatment and later rechristened REBT in 1992. Ellis continued to use REBT until his death in 2007.

The ABC Model

Ellis suggested that individuals wrongly condemn external occasions for unhappiness. He said, nevertheless, that it is our analysis of these events that really exists at the heart of our emotional distress. To explain this process, Ellis developed what he referred to as the ABC Model:

A– Activating Event: Something happens in the environment around you.

B– Beliefs: You hold an idea about the occasion or situation.

C– Consequence: You have an emotional feedback to your idea.

The occasions and situations that individuals experience throughout life are only one piece of the problem. In order to understand the effect of such events, it is also essential to check out the beliefs individuals hold regarding these experiences in addition to the feelings that arise as a result of those ideas.

The Basic Steps

In order to better comprehend exactly how REBT looks, it is important to take a more detailed check out the healing procedure itself.

Identify the Underlying Irrational Thought Patterns and also Beliefs.

The very first step at the same time is to identify the irrational thoughts, sensations, and also ideas that bring about mental distress. Oftentimes, these unreasonable beliefs are reflected as absolutes, as in "I must," "I should," or "I cannot." According to Ellis, several of the most typical irrational beliefs consist of:

Really feeling exceedingly upset over other individuals' blunders or transgression.

Thinking that you need to be 100 percent successful as well as proficient in everything to be valued and rewarding.

If you avoid life's obstacles or troubles, thinking that you will be happier.

Really feeling that you have no control over your own happiness; that your contentment and also joy are dependent upon outside forces.

By holding such stubborn ideas, it ends up being practically difficult to reply to situations in an emotionally healthy method. Possessing such rigid assumptions of ourselves and others only results in frustration, regret, recrimination, as well as stress and anxiety.

Challenge the Irrational Beliefs

Once these underlying feelings have been identified, the next action is to test these misconceptions. In order to do this, the therapist should contest these ideas utilizing also confrontational and also very straight techniques.

Ellis suggested that rather than merely being encouraging and also warm, the specialist needs to be blunt, sincere, as well as rational in order to press individuals toward changing their actions as well as ideas.

Gain Insight as well as Recognize Irrational Thought Patterns

As you might imagine, REBT can be a daunting procedure for the customer. Dealing with irrational thought patterns can be challenging, particularly since approving these beliefs as harmful is far from very easy. As soon as the client has actually determined the bothersome beliefs, the procedure of in fact changing these ideas can be a lot more challenging.

While it is perfectly typical to feel upset when you make a blunder, the objective of logical emotive habits therapy is to help people react logically to such circumstances. When encountered with this kind of situation in the future, the psychologically healthy action would certainly be to realize that while it would certainly be fantastic to be ideal as well as never ever make mistakes, it is not practical to anticipate success in every endeavor.

It is additionally crucial to acknowledge that while sensible emotive behavior therapy utilizes cognitive strategies to aid customers, it additionally focuses on feelings as well as habits also. In addition to recognizing and disputing irrational ideas, clients and also therapists also interact to target the psychological reactions that come with troublesome thoughts. Customers are additionally motivated to alter unwanted actions using such points as reflection, journaling, as well as guided imagery.

Cognitive Therapy

This kind of treatment is fixated identifying as well as transforming imprecise or altered reasoning patterns, psychological reactions, and also behaviors.

Cognitive Distortions

What's a cognitive distortion as well as why do so many people have them? Cognitive distortions are just ways that our mind persuades us of something that isn't actually true. These incorrect ideas are typically made use of to strengthen negative attitude or emotions– informing ourselves points that sound precise as well as rational, but truly just serve to keep us really feeling negative concerning ourselves.

The individual is just seeing points in absolutes– that if they fall short at one thing, they must fall short at all points. If they included, "I need to be a full loser and also failing" to their reasoning, that would additionally be an example of overgeneralization– taking a failure at one particular task and generalizing it their very self and identification.

Cognitive distortions go to the core of what several cognitive-behavioral and also other sort of specialists assist a person and attempt discover to change in psychotherapy. By learning to appropriately recognize this type of "stinkin' thinkin'," an individual can then address the negative thinking back, as well as refute it. By shooting down the negative thinking over and over once again, it will gradually reduce overtime and also be immediately changed by more reasonable, balanced thinking.

The Most Common Cognitive Distortions

In 1976, psychologist Aaron Beck first suggested the concept behind cognitive distortions. Also in the 1980s, David Burns was in charge of popularizing it with typical names and examples for the distortions.

1. Filtering system

Individual engaging in filter (or "mental filtering system) takes the negative details and also magnifies those details while straining all positive aspects of a circumstance. As an example, an individual may pick out solitary, unpleasant information, and also harp on it specifically to make sure that their vision of fact comes to be distorted or darkened. When a cognitive filter is applied, the person sees only the adverse and also disregards anything favorable.

2. Polarized Thinking (or "Black and also White" Thinking)

A person with polarized assuming areas individuals or circumstances in "either/or" groups, with no tones of grey or enabling for the intricacy of many people and also a lot of situations. A person with black-and-white thinking sees things only in extremes.

3. Overgeneralization

In this cognitive distortion, a person involves a basic conclusion based upon a single occurrence or a single item of evidence. If something bad takes place simply once, they expect it to occur over and over once more. A person might see a single, unpleasant occasion as part of a continuous pattern of defeat.

For instance, if a student gets an inadequate quality on one paper in one semester, they end they are a horrible student as well as must quit college.

4. Jumping to Conclusions.

Without individuals saying so, a person who leaps to conclusions knows what one more person is really feeling as well as believing– and also exactly why they act the means they do. Specifically, an individual has the ability to figure out how others are really feeling toward the person, as though they might read their mind. Leaping to conclusions can additionally materialize itself as fortune-telling, where a person thinks their whole future is pre-ordained (whether it be in school, job, or romantic partnerships).

A person may assume that another person is holding an animosity versus them, yet does not actually trouble to find out if they are correct. Another example entailing fortune-telling is when a person may expect that things will turn out badly in their next connection, as well as will really feel convinced that their forecast is already a well-known fact, so why trouble dating.

5. Catastrophizing

When a person participates in catastrophizing, they anticipate disaster to strike. This is additionally described as magnifying, and also can additionally come out in its contrary actions, minimizing. In this distortion, an individual reads about an issue as well as utilizes suppose inquiries (e.g., "What if misfortune strikes?" "What if it takes place to me?") to imagine the absolute worst taking place.

For instance, a person could overemphasize the relevance of unimportant occasions (such as their error, or another person's accomplishment). Or they might wrongly diminish the size of substantial events up until they show up little (for example, a person's very own preferable qualities or someone else's imperfections).

With method, you can learn to answer each of these cognitive distortions.

6. Personalization.

Personalization is a distortion where an individual thinks that everything others state or do is some kind of direct, personal response to them. A person who experiences this kind of assuming will also compare themselves to others, trying to establish who is smarter; far better looking, and so on

. An individual involving in customization might also see themselves as the reason of some harmful external occasion that they were not accountable for.

7. Control Fallacies

This distortion entails two (2) related however different beliefs regarding remaining in complete control of every scenario in an individual's life. In the initial, if we feel on the surface managed, we see ourselves as powerless a sufferer of destiny. As an example, "I cannot aid it if the quality of the job is poor. My manager required I work overtime on it."

The misconception of inner control has us thinking obligation for the discomfort and joy of every person around us. For example, "Why aren't you satisfied? Is it as a result of something I did?"

8. Fallacy of Fairness

In the fallacy of justness, an individual really feels resentful since they assume that they know what is fair, however, other individuals will not agree with them. As our parents inform us when we're maturing and also something doesn't go our way, "Life isn't constantly reasonable." Individuals that undergo life applying a measuring ruler against every situation judging its "fairness" will certainly typically feel resentful, angry, and even pessimism as a result of it. Due to the fact that life isn't fair—points will not always exercise in a person's favor, even when they should.

9. Criticizing

When an individual participates in criticizing, they hold other people in charge of their psychological pain. They may additionally take the opposite track and also instead condemn themselves for each issue– also those clearly outside their very own control.

"Stop making me really feel negative regarding myself!" No one can "make" us feel any kind of certain way– we only have control over our emotional responses and also own feelings.

10. Should

Should declarations (" I ought to pick up after myself extra ...") appear as a list of uncompromising guidelines regarding exactly how everyone need to act. People that damage the regulations make an individual complying with these must declarations upset. They likewise really feel guilty when they violate their very own guidelines. An individual may frequently believe they are trying to inspire themselves with "shoulds "and "must've," as if they have to be punished prior to they can do anything.

The emotional consequence is guilt: When a person directs should statements toward others, they often feel resentment, anger and frustration.

11. Emotional Reasoning.

The distortion of emotional thinking can be summed up by the declaration, "If I really feel in this way, it has to be true." Whatever a person is feeling is believed to be true immediately as well as unconditionally. They must be stupid and boring if a person feels stupid and boring.

Feelings are exceptionally solid in people, and can void our rational thoughts and reasoning. Psychological thinking is when an individual's emotions takes control of our assuming completely, removing all rationality as well as reasoning. The person who participates in psychological thinking assumes that their harmful feelings show the means points really are– "I feel it, for that reason it should be true.".

12. Fallacy of Change

In the misconception of modification, a person anticipates that other people will alter to match them if they simply pressure or cajole them enough. Because their hopes for success and happiness seem to depend entirely on them, a person needs to change people.

This distortion is often located in thinking around connections. For example, girlfriend who tries to get her boyfriend to improve his appearance and manners, in the belief that this boyfriend is perfect in every other way and will make them happy if they only changed these few minor things.

13. Global Labeling

In Global Labeling (likewise referred to as mislabeling), a person generalizes one or two top qualities right into an adverse global judgment regarding themselves or another individual. This is a severe form of over generalizing. Rather than describing an error in context of a details circumstance, a person will affix an unhealthy global label to themselves or others.

For example, they may claim, "I'm a loser" in a situation where they fell short at a specific job. When another person's habits massages a person the wrong way– without troubling to comprehend any kind of context around why– they may attach an unhealthy label to him, such as "He's a genuine jerk.".

Mislabeling involves defining an occasion with language that is very colored as well as mentally packed. For instance, as opposed to stating a person drops her children off at daycare daily, an individual that is mislabeling may state that "She deserts her children to complete strangers."

14. Always Being Right

When a person takes part in this distortion, they are consistently putting other people on trial to confirm that their own opinions and actions are the absolute appropriate ones. To a person engaging in "always being right," being wrong is unthinkable– they will certainly most likely to any kind of size to demonstrate their rightness.

"I don't care how badly arguing with me makes you feel, I'm going to win this argument no matter what because I'm right." Being right often is more vital than the feelings of others around a person who takes part in this cognitive distortion, also loved ones.

15. Paradise's Reward Fallacy.

The last cognitive distortion is the fallacy that a person's sacrifice as well as self-denial will at some point pay off, as if some global force is keeping rating. This is a riff on the fallacy of fairness, due to the fact that in a reasonable globe, the people that work the hardest will certainly obtain the largest incentive. A person who sacrifices as well as works hard yet does not experience the anticipated resolve, will usually feel bitter when the incentive does not come.

How Do You Fix Cognitive Distortions?

So, now that you recognize what cognitive distortions are, just how do you tackle them? The bright side is that you can fix your illogical thinking, and also we can aid you do that

Cognitive distortions have a way of playing chaos with our lives if we let them. A cognitive distortion takes area in our minds when we experience a distressing event in our lives– a difference at job, a debate with a partner, a poor outcome in college– and also we believe concerning it in a means that strengthens negativity as well as feeling bad.

Cognitive distortions– also called "stinkin' thinkin'"– can be undone, however it takes effort and great deals of technique, daily. If you wish to stop the illogical thinking, you can start by experimenting with the workouts listed below.

Exactly How to Fix Common Cognitive Distortions

You can utilize any one or a mix of the approaches described below to combat unreasonable, cognitive distortions and also automatic ideas. Attempt a few of them out and also try to find the one that appears to function best for you, since different people reply to different ways of repairing their irrational ideas.

1. Recognize the Cognitive Distortion

One of the most important action of repairing any type of problem in your life is recognizing exactly what the problem is and also how comprehensive it is in your life. A grease monkey begins with an analysis of your cars and truck when it has a trouble.

In this very same fashion, you require to recognize as well as track the cognitive distortions in your day-to-day reasoning initially, before you start working to change them. You do this by developing a list of the frustrating thoughts throughout the day, as you're having them. This will certainly enable you to examine them later for suits with a listing of cognitive distortions.

An assessment of your cognitive distortions allows you to see which distortions that you find intriguing. Furthermore, this procedure allows you to think about each issue or situation in an extra all-natural or practical manner. David Burns called this workout keeping a daily state of mind log, yet nowadays you can use an app or anything that's convenient to tape-record your cognitive distortions.

2. Examine the Evidence

Just like a judge overseeing a test, the next action is to eliminate yourself from the emotionality of the upsetting event or episode of irrational thinking in order to analyze the evidence extra objectively. A comprehensive evaluation of an experience allows you to identify the basis for your altered ideas. You ought to determine a number of experiences and also scenarios where you had success if you are excessively self-critical.

One effective technique for taking a look at the proof is to look at private ideas attached to the event, and also objectively choose whether those declarations reflect a viewpoint or truth. Segregating truths from point of views can help you establish which are likely to be an element of a cognitive distortion (the viewpoints) and consequently need your focus as well as efforts to undo.

3. Double Standard Method

A choice to "self-talk" that is undermining and also rough is to speak to ourselves in the exact same compassionate and also caring manner in which we would certainly talk with a pal in a comparable circumstance. We are often much harder on ourselves than the people we care about in our lives, whether it be a good friend or relative. We would certainly never consider talking to a close friend in the way we talk to ourselves in our own mind.

Rather than treating yourself with a various criterion than what you hold every person else to, why not make use of one single criterion for every person including yourself? Isn't that more reasonable than utilizing a double-standard? Provide yourself the same support that you would a trusted close friend.

These are the very same kinds of ideas that run via several pupils' minds prior to a test. Can you respond to such automated, unfavorable thoughts back with a reasonable response? "You're going to do well on this examination, I just understand it.

4. Believing in Shades of Gray

Finding out to undo black-and-white (or polarized) reasoning can be difficult, since our minds take cognitive shortcuts to streamline handling of stimulations in order to rush our ability to decide or pick an action. Black-and-white reasoning can in some cases serve a good function, however it typically leads an individual down a path of illogical idea also.

As opposed to considering a trouble or circumstance in an either-or polarity, assuming in shades of gray requires us to examine points on a scale of 0 to100. When a plan or goal is not fully realized, consider as well as assess the experience as a partial success on this sort of range.

Somebody could believe, "You cannot do anything. You simply blew your diet plan by having that second bite of ice cream." What is the probability that an individual's entire dieting routine– that they've been following rigorously for months– is now made useless by a solitary added bite of ice cream? On our range of 0 with 100, it might be about a one percent possibility.

5. Experimental Method

Can you examine whether your unreasonable thoughts have any kind of basis actually outside of a trial? You sure can – by utilizing the very same kinds of methods that science makes use of in order to evaluate a theory.

Let's say you've been putting off organizing your digital photos because it'll be "too hard" or "I just can't do it." What if the task was broken down right into smaller sized components, such as tackling simply a solitary month each time in one sitting? Is the idea that it's simply "also difficult" still true, since you've broken the task right into smaller sized, attainable parts?

In one more instance, think of an individual who believes with time that she is no longer liked as by her close friends due to the fact that they never ever get in touch with her on social networks or call. Could that individual examination whether it held true that her friends no longer like her? What if she connected to them as well as asked them out to lunch or for drinks eventually? While it's not likely all of her close friends will accept an invitation, it's likely at the very least one or two of them will, providing clear evidence in support of the fact that her close friends still like her.

6. Survey Method

Similar to the speculative method, the survey technique is concentrated on asking others in a similar circumstance about their experiences to figure out just how unreasonable our thoughts could be. Utilizing this method, an individual looks for the point of views of others relating to whether their thoughts and also attitudes are reasonable.

A person might believe that romantic partners should never fight. That person would soon realize that all couples fight, and while it may be a good idea not to go to bed angry, plenty of people do, and their relationship is just fine despite that.

Check in with a few trusted friends to see what their opinions and experiences are if you want to double-check on the rationality of your thought.

7. The Semantic Method

When a person takes part in a collection of must statements (" I should do this" or "I should not do that"), they are applying a collection of customs to their behavior that might make little sense to others. Should statements suggest a judgment concerning your or another person's behavior– one that might be even hurtful and unhelpful.

Whenever you find yourself using a should declaration, attempt substituting "It would certainly be nice if ..." instead. This semantic difference can work wonders in your very own mind, as you quit "should-ing" yourself to fatality as well as start looking at the globe in a different, much more positive fashion. "Shoulds" make a person feel negative and regret regarding themselves. "Wouldn't it behave and also healthier if I began enjoying what I consumed more?" This places the assumed into an extra curious, analytical phrasing– one where the solution might be of course, but could likewise be no (for instance, if you've simply begun cancer cells therapy, currently it's not a good time to transform your consuming habits).

8. Interpretations

For people who are more intellectual as well as like to say regarding minutiae, this technique of arguing with your cognitive distortions can be found to be inconvenient. What does it suggest to specify ourselves as "substandard," "a loser," "a fool," or "uncommon." An evaluation of these as well as other worldwide tags might disclose that they much more carefully stand for particular behaviors, or a recognizable actions pattern, instead of the complete person.

When a person starts delving into the definition of a label and asking questions about those definitions, the results can be surprising. What does it mean to think of yourself as "inferior"? What are their specific work experiences and backgrounds?

9. Re-attribution

In customization as well as criticizing cognitive distortions, an individual will certainly blame to themselves for all of the negative things they experience, no matter what the actual cause.

In re-attribution, an individual recognizes exterior elements as well as other people that contributed to the trouble or event. No matter the degree of responsibility an individual assumes, a person's energy is ideal used in the pursuit of resolutions to troubles or identifying ways to deal with situations. By assigning duty as necessary, you're not attempting to deflect blame, but guarantee you're not condemning yourself entirely for something that wasn't totally your fault.

As an example, if a project at the workplace needs to be done promptly and also you was among the members of the 5-member group, you're one-fifth responsible for the task missing its due date. From an unbiased point of view, you are not entirely to blame for the missed out on deadline.

10. Cost-Benefit Analysis

This technique for addressing an irrational belief relies upon inspiration instead of realities to help a person reverse the cognitive distortion. In this strategy, it is helpful to note the benefits as well as downsides of sensations, ideas, and also actions. A cost-benefit evaluation will assist to determine what a person is getting from feeling negative, distorted reasoning, and also inappropriate behavior.

"How will it assist me to think this adverse, irrational idea, as well as just how will it hurt me?" You'll find it easier to talk back and refute the irrational belief if you find the disadvantages of believing a thought outweigh the advantages.

Multimodal Therapy

This type of CBT suggests that mental problems need to be dealt with by addressing seven (7) interconnected yet various techniques, which are habits, influence, sensation, images, cognition, social aspects and drug/biological factors to consider.

Often referred to as merely MMT, multimodal treatment is a diverse kind of psychotherapy. Eclectic therapies attract from as well as integrate components of numerous disciplines, psychology theories, or restorative approaches.

Initially, a behavior specialist and also leader in the area of cognitive behavioral therapy (CBT), Arnold Lazarus noted that numerous people treated with traditional CBT for clinical depression, stress and anxiety conditions, and other problems ended up relapsing at some point. They had actually been treated with what he called "slim band" treatment, when what they truly required was a "broad-spectrum" therapy approach.

In order to address this inadequacy in various other types of psychotherapy– and also to guarantee a much more efficient and also thorough technique to treatment– Lazarus created the BASIC I.D. This principle plays a central duty in multimodal therapy.

The BASIC I.D.

Multimodal treatment is based on the premise that seven related but distinctive dimensions or "techniques" of psychological performance, temperament, and also individuality are analyzed and addressed in therapy. These have actually come to be understood by the phrase "BASIC ID". These 7 methods are:

- Actions
- Influence
- Sensation
- Imagery
- Cognition
- Interpersonal
- Drugs/Health/Biology

Habits represents whatever an individual does–actions, practices, gestures, etc. Behaviors can be undesirable or healthy and balanced, harmful or useful, ethical or unethical, mature or childlike, suitable or unsuitable, law-abiding or unlawful, uncontrollable, impulsive, or managed, and so on. Many individuals seek treatment to transform unwanted habits that are triggering troubles in their life such as overeating, nail-biting, hoarding, acting out, self-mutilating, or alcohol consumption exceedingly. Traditional behavior therapy focuses on transforming the habits itself with using techniques such as modeling, aversive conditioning, and organized desensitization. Sadly, practically every unwanted behavior is connected to and also interacting with other techniques too, such as experience, cognition, and emotion. When those aren't addressed as well, regression usually occurs.

One of the major reasons individuals seek treatment is because they do not such as the way they really

feel. Even those who seek therapy for other factors–
e.g. to shed weight, save their marriage, or
overcome a phobia– the underlying inspiration is
almost constantly to alter the method they feel
mentally.

Experience relate to our detects– sight, hearing,
touch, preference, and also smell– and all of our
physical experiences. Examples of sensations
include muscle stress, knots in the stomach,
"butterflies," physical discomfort, competing heart,
tension frustrations, chilly hands, creeping skin,
lack of breath, sweating, and nausea or vomiting.
Hallucinations as well as impressions are likewise
examples of feelings.

Experience is just one of the methods that is most
often disregarded in psychotherapy, even though an
unpleasant sensation can be very unpleasant.
Feelings can supply a lot of useful information in
treatment. For instance, unsettled injury often
materializes in psychosomatic signs and symptoms
that may be misinterpreted by the client, leading
him or her to seek medical treatment instead. Many
people attempt to resolve unpleasant sensations
with medicine or other compounds (e.g. alcohol or
medications).

Images refers to the mental images and images
individuals produce in their mind– in other words,

what they picture fantasize, as well as daydream around. An individual's self-image would fall under this group. Individuals that struggle with anxiousness often feed their anxiety with overstated, fearfulimagesof things that might take place in the future. People with depression often paint extremely adverse, distorted images in their mind. Those fighting eating disorders have distorted body images that play a considerable duty in their problems. Learning to change one's mental imagery can go a long way towards causing desired adjustments.

Cognition refers to thoughts (inclusive of believed patterns), attitudes, judgments, as well as ideas. Adverse thoughts, including adverse "self-talk" and also limiting or altered beliefs almost always play a substantial duty in depression, stress and anxiety, as well as other disorders. Deeply deep-rooted beliefs about not being deserving or deserving, for example, can undermine an individual's relationships and also level of success in life if those beliefs are never ever effectively dealt with.

Interpersonal refers to individuals' connections with others, as well as their social abilities– i.e., how they relate to and interact with people normally. Many individuals seek therapy to attend to connection issues, such as dealing with a separation or fixing conflict with a liked one.

Others look for therapy since they've ended up being isolated or feel detached.

Medications, health and wellness, and biology fit to form the seventh modality. This method encompasses numerous points, including physical health and wellness (e.g. ailment, health and wellness conditions, physical limitations, age-related health and wellness issues, chronic discomfort), organic factors (e.g. mind chemistry or genetics), as well as the demand for drug or other types of clinical/organic therapy. Also consisted of in this modality are way of living routines that influence one's health, such as exercise (or do not have thereof), diet regimen and also nourishment, rest habits, alcohol, overindulging and also medicine use, cigarette smoking routines, and so on

. In multimodal therapy, these seven modalities are analyzed by the specialist in two (2) ways– by speaking with the client and by having him or her fill out a questionnaire referred to as the Multimodal Life History Inventory.

Multimodal Life History Inventory.

This inventory is usually completed by the customer at home, adhering to the initial session. It is 15 pages long and consists of the following sections:

General Information– This section consists of name, address, day of birth, marriage standing, current and also previous work, living scenario, and so on. It additionally asks about personal and also family history of self-destruction efforts, as well as any type of family history of psychological health issue.

Personal and also Social History– In addition to fundamental inquiries concerning parents as well as siblings, this area additionally asks about parents personalities, attitudes, and also methods of punishment, the client's connection with both parents, home setting growing up, education (including scholastic strengthand also weak points), and issues that took place during childhood years (e.g. bullying, sexual abuse, substance abuse, medical concerns, lack of friends, and so on).

Description of Presenting Problem– This area asks the customer to define his/her primary issues, level of seriousness, when they started, what the customer has attempted, etc.

. Assumptions Concerning Therapy– This area asks the customer to document what she or he thinks of therapy, including how long it needs to last as well as what characteristics an excellent specialist should have.

Method Analysis of Current Problems– This area enables the customer to provide more extensive details regarding the troubles that led him or her to treatment. It covers the seven modalities in the BASIC I.D. with a mix of questions, fill-in-the-blank statements, rating scales, and lists for every technique. This is the longest section of the survey, and is fairly detailed in its range.

The last web page of the supply allows the client to explain any type of considerable experiences or memories (from youth or any other time in the person's life) that he or she really feels the specialist must know about.

When the specialist has actually evaluated the customer's seven techniques– the BASIC I.D.– she or he will determine the most effective healing methods as well as techniques to resolve them, starting with whichever method is the most troublesome.

Even though policies and strategies play an essential role in MMT, the partnership between therapist and customer is likewise very vital. Clients list the qualities of the "ideal" specialist (in their eyes) on the inventory. Multimodal specialists acknowledge the value of adjusting their partnership design depending on the customer's requirements as well as preferences (info that can usually be acquired from the stock).

Some customers do a lot better with a specialist who is extremely cozy, personable, and also understanding. In addition, some customers choose working with a specialist who is really energetic and also straight, while others choose a therapist that listens really well and takes a less direct strategy.

Common Techniques Used in MMT

The strategies as well as approaches made use of by the specialist originated from many different psychotherapeutic methods along with other disciplines, consisting of Gestalt therapy, timeless behavior therapy, cognitive treatment, home therapy, psychodrama, logotherapy, assisted images, bibliotherapy, anger administration, leisure training, hypnotherapy, biofeedback, and also social skills training to name several. Specialists are motivated to use methods that are empirically supported as high as possible. Sometimes, the therapist might need to refer customers to an additional company.

Actions

- Modelling

- Self-monitoring

- Systematic desensitization

- Reinforcement

- Contingency agreements

- Response rate

- Shame assaulting

- Paradoxical intention

- Behavior rehearsal

Affect

- Emotion guideline

- Anger monitoring

- Feeling recognition

- Pleasant task schedule

- Identify triggers

Feeling

- Biofeedback

- Relaxation training

- Massage therapy

- Hypnosis

- Meditation

- Sensate focus training

- Yoga

Imagery

- Mastery images

- Positive imagery

- Aversive imagery

- Time estimate imagery

- Thought stopping imagery

- Coping imagery

- Anti-future shock imagery

Cognitive

- Cognitive restructuring

- Positive self-talk

- Thought documents

- Disputing irrational beliefs

- Thought quitting

- Bibliotherapy

Interpersonal

- Assertiveness training

- Social abilities training

- Intimacy training

- Communication abilities training

- Role turnaround

- Fixed role therapy

Drugs/ Health/ Biology

- Exercise

- Smoking cessation program

- Weight management

- Nutrition education and learning

- Lifestyle changes

- Consult with medical professional or various other doctor (with customer's consent)

- Refer to professionals

Problems, Conditions, and also Problems that Can Benefit from MMT.

Adhering to are simply several of the problems and also problems that might benefit from multimodal therapy:

- Depression

- Generalized anxiousness disorder

- PTSD

- Eating conditions

- Panic problem

- Social anxiety condition

- Relationship issues

- Weight problems

- Emotional eating

- Stress monitoring

- Behavioral issues

- Compulsive habits

- Low self-worth

- Insomnia

- Chronic discomfort

Benefits of Multimodal Therapy.

While no treatment is best, multimodal therapy has numerous advantages that deserve taking into consideration.Multimodal treatment is a very thorough and also flexible type of psychiatric therapy. Its "broad-spectrum" strategy to therapy is just one of the reasons it's so very effective.

The comprehensive assessment that plays an essential function in MMT helps ensure an extra exact medical diagnosis as well as likewise helps the therapist select extremely focused treatment approaches. With each other, these two elements improve the efficiency of treatment and increase the likeliness of long-lasting outcomes.

In MMT, therapy is tailored to the client's demands by utilizing a mix of techniques and approaches from many different therapeutic techniques as well as disciplines. The specialist meticulously chooses the ones that are appropriate for the particular client and most likely to be the most reliable. Since the methods aren't limited to a specific mental theory or positioning, the range of potential interventions at the specialist's disposal is a lot broader than in various other types of psychotherapy.

Multimodal treatment addresses the seven crucial modalities of individuality and working, as well as recognizes which ones are one of the most problematic. This makes certain that no technique is forgotten, which would make the client vulnerable to relapse.

Multimodal treatment thinks about the truth that customers' troubles normally include a communication of a number of modalities as opposed to simply a couple of.

By examining a customer's BASIC I.D. and also attending to one of the most troublesome locations with appropriate treatments, MMT helps the customer make positive modifications that align more carefully with his or her suitable self.

Specialists that make use of multimodal therapy don't just tailor the strategies as well as interventions to their clients; they additionally tailor their restorative design to fit the client's demands– i.e. the customer's specific manner of reasoning and also feeling. Collaborating with a client in a design that suits him or her normally enhances the therapeutic connection, which is a crucial element of reliable treatment.

Multimodal Therapy in Practice

You may still be a bit uncertain as to just how all the pieces fit together in terms of exactly how MMT really functions if you've reviewed this far. Complying with is an instance of the way multimodal treatment could be made use of to address a client that has problems with psychological eating.

Behavior: Remove home cooking from the house and also workplace; make a listing of option, healthy behaviors you can do when negative feelings develop (e.g. choose a stroll, call a pal, or write in a journal), as well as select one to do each time you really feel lured to comfort yourself with foods.

Affect: Use tension administration techniques to reduced tension; recognize psychological triggers that cause comforting yourself with food– i.e. what feelings (e.g. rage, unhappiness, dullness) often tend to be present when you feel the requirement to self-soothe with food?

Sensation: Use leisure approaches to manage and decrease stress and anxiety.

Imagery: Visualize yourself handling problem and various other stressors smoothly and effectively.

Cognition: Keep a journal of the negative ideas that result in emotional consuming (i.e. what are you informing yourself just before you reach for the bag of cookies?); use constructive self-talk when tempted to eat for comfort.

Interpersonal: Seek assistance from good friends or family when you're experiencing extreme adverse feelings; technique assertiveness abilities in order to minimize sensations of powerlessness as well as inferiority that trigger emotional eating.

Medications/ health and wellness/ biology: Get some type of exercise every day to help reduce tension; obtain enough rest so you're well-rested every day (as exhaustion makes adverse feelings also worse).

Additional instance, for somebody taking care of depression:

Habits: Keep a normal sleep timetable; do a minimum of one satisfying task a day, even if you don't feel like it.

Affect: Reduce sadness by searching for the happiness in small things; reveal negative feelings in treatment and also/ or writing in a journal as opposed to maintaining them inside.

Feeling: Use yoga or massage treatment to reduce muscular tissue stress.

Images: Visualize a favorable, beneficial future when bleak pictures enter your mind.

Cognition: Practice favorable self-talk; jot down unfavorable beliefs that are contributing to feelings of unimportance as well as sadness; test their precision.

Interpersonal: Avoid seclusion by invest more time with individuals you enjoy or engaging in tasks that entail interacting with other people.

Medicines/wellness/biology: Exercise frequently to improve mood; take antidepressant drug to aid ease symptoms as well as enhance general functioning.

The interventions made use of above are just instances of what could be used, yet many other treatments as well as techniques could be utilized in their location relying on the certain client as well as his or her BASIC I.D. The specialist may utilize totally different methods than those above to attend to the exact same fundamental issue with an additional customer, relying on multiple factors. This is among the toughness of MMT– it's not a cookie-cutter/ one-size-fits-all approach. Instead, the treatment is meticulously customized to fit the client's needs, based on the details gotten from the initial interview as well as the Multimodal Life History Inventory.

Contraindications for Multimodal Therapy

People that are psychotic, manic, or actively suicidal aren't going to be appropriate for this treatment strategy. It would certainly additionally be impossible, or at the very least incredibly hard, for such people to complete the Multimodal Life History Inventory, considering that doing so calls for the capacity to sit still, focus, and also believe clearly.

An additional contraindication for MMT is active drug abuse. It can be properly utilized for individuals that are in healing, either as part of a dual diagnosis therapy program (in which mental health and wellness concerns and also substance abuse or addiction are dealt with concurrently) or adhering to drug and alcohol therapy when the person is sober as well as tidy. Nevertheless, when somebody is actively using alcohol and medicines, psychotherapy of any type of kind will certainly have very restricted– if any kind of– advantage.

DIALECTICAL BEHAVIOR THERAPY

This type of cognitive-behavioral treatment addresses assuming habits and patterns and also incorporates approaches such as psychological law and mindfulness.

Dialectical behavior therapy (DBT) is a kind of cognitive behavior modification. Its main objectives are to teach people how to live in the minute, cope healthily with anxiety, control feelings, as well as improve partnerships with others.

It was initially meant for individuals with borderline personality disorder (BPD) but has actually considering that been adapted for other conditions where the person exhibits self-destructive behavior, such as consuming problems and also chemical abuse. It is additionally in some cases used to treat trauma.

DBT is originated from a thoughtful procedure called dialectics. Dialectics is based on the idea that everything is made up of revers and that change takes place when one opposing pressure is stronger than the various other, or in more academic terms–antithesis, thesis, as well as synthesis.

A lot more especially, dialectics makes three standard assumptions:

- All points are adjoined.

- Change is consistent and also unpreventable.

- Opposites can be integrated to form a closer estimate of the reality.

In DBT, the client and therapist are functioning to settle the seeming opposition in between self-acceptance as well as modification in order to produce positive modifications in the patient.

An additional strategy offered by Linehan as well as her coworkers was validation. Linehan and her team found that with recognition, in addition to the promote change, patients were more likely to cooperate and less most likely to suffer distress at the concept of change. The therapist validates that the individual's actions "make sense" within the context of his individual experiences without always concurring that they are the best approach to resolving the problem.

How It Works

DBT has currently progressed right into a conventional sort of cognitive behavior modification. When an individual is going through DBT, they can anticipate to join three restorative setups:

A classroom where a person is taught behavioral abilities by doing research assignments and also role-playing brand-new methods of interacting with individuals. Generally, the class fulfills for two to three hours on a regular basis.

Specific treatment with a qualified specialist where those found out behavioral abilities are adjusted to a person's personal life obstacles. Running simultaneously with the classroom assignment, specific therapy sessions generally last for 60 minutes, when a week.

Phone training in which an individual can call their therapist in between sessions to obtain support on handling a difficult at-the-moment circumstance.

In DBT, private specialists likewise meet a consultation group to help them remain inspired in treating their patients and also help them navigate hard and intricate concerns.

While each restorative setup has its very own collection structure and objectives, the complying with features of DBT are discovered in group abilities training, individual psychotherapy, and also phone coaching:

Assistance: You'll be encouraged to identify your favorable toughness and attributes and also establish and also utilize them.

Behavioral: You'll find out to assess any kind of trouble or devastating habits patterns as well as replace them with effective and healthy ones.

Cognitive: You'll concentrate on transforming ideas and also ideas, as well as habits, or actions that are not effective or practical.

Ability: You'll discover brand-new skills to boost your capacities.

Approval and modification: You'll find out approaches to approve and also tolerate your life, emotions, and yourself in addition to abilities to assist you make positive changes in your actions as well as interactions with others.

Partnership: You'll find out to communicate effectively as well as work together as a group (specialist, group specialist, psychoanalyst).

DBT Strategies

Individuals going through DBT are shown how to efficiently alter their habits making use of four major approaches:

Core Mindfulness

These skills will certainly aid you to reduce down so you can concentrate on healthy and balanced coping skills in the middle of psychological discomfort. Mindfulness can aid you to stay tranquil and also avoid involving in automatic adverse thought patterns and also spontaneous actions.

Test Exercise: Observe Mindfulness Skill

Take notice of your breath. Make note of the feeling of breathing out as well as breathing in, observing your belly rise and fall as you breathe.

Distress Tolerance

Distress tolerance teaches you to approve yourself and also the current situation. More particularly, you discover how to tolerate or endure crises utilizing four techniques: disturbance, self-soothing, boosting the motion, and also thinking about pros and cons. By learning distress tolerance strategies, you'll have the ability to prepare ahead of time for any kind of intense feelings as well as handle them with a more favorable long-term outlook.

Taste Exercise: Putting Your Body in Charge

Go down the stairways. Go outside if you're inside. Get up and also stroll around if you're sitting. The idea is to distract yourself by enabling your feelings to follow your body.

Interpersonal Effectiveness

Interpersonal effectiveness assists you to end up being extra assertive in a relationship (as an example, sharing requirements as well as saying "no") while still keeping that partnership favorable as well as healthy and balanced. This occurs by learning to pay attention as well as communicate effectively, handle challenging individuals, and regard yourself and also others.

Experience Exercise: GIVE

Use the phrase GIVE to improve partnerships as well as favorable interaction:

- Gentle: Don't strike, endanger, or judge

- Interest: Show interest with good listening skills (don't disturb when talking).

- Validate: Acknowledge the person's ideas and feelings.

- Easy: Try to have a very easy attitude (smile and stay light-hearted).

Emotion Regulation.

Feeling regulation offers a set of skills that aid to maintain your psychological system healthy and balanced and working. It educates you to readjust your emotions, including the intensity, when you have it, and also just how you react to it. By acknowledging and coping with adverse feelings (for instance, anger), you can decrease your emotional vulnerability and also have much more positive emotional experiences.

Taste Exercise: Opposite Action.

Recognize exactly how you're feeling as well as do the contrary. Do the contrary if you're sad as well as feel like taking out from close friends as well as home. Make strategies to see friends and family as well as stay social.

Is DBT Right for You?

While the majority of research to day has actually focused on the efficiency of DBT for individuals with borderline personality disorder, along with co-occurring thoughts of self-destruction and also self-harm, post-traumatic stress disorder, and also compound use disorders, DBT has also been shown to help a selection of psychological health problems including:.

- ADHD

- Binge eating condition

- Bipolar disorder

- Bulimia

- Generalized anxiety condition

- Major depressive (consisting of treatment-resistant significant clinical depression and chronic depression).

- Post-traumatic tension disorder

- Substance use disorder

- Suicidal as well as self-harming actions

Researchers have actually additionally located that DBT works regardless of age, gender, sexual preference, and also race/ethnicity.

While each kind of cognitive-behavioral treatment provides its own special strategy, each fixate addressing the underlying idea patterns that contribute to psychological distress.

Individual cognitive behavioral therapy

A psychologist will work with the child to improve:

Anger management skills

Anger is an extremely effective sensation that can occur when you are distressed, wounded, irritated, or disappointed. If you hold your anger inside, it can lead to passive-aggressive behavior like "obtaining back" at people without informing them why or being hostile and also essential.

Recognizing rage:

Rage is a normal, healthy emotion, neither great neither poor. While it's flawlessly regular to really feel upset when you've been mistreated or wronged, rage becomes a problem when you express it in a way that hurts yourself or others.

You could think that venting your anger is healthy and balanced, that individuals around you are too sensitive, that your rage is warranted, or that you need to show your fierceness to get respect. The fact is that temper is a lot more likely to have a negative impact on the means people see you, impair your judgment, as well as get in the method of success.

Impacts of anger

Chronic rage that flares up constantly or spirals out of hand can have significant consequences for your:

Physical health. Constantly operating at high levels of tension and also anger makes you a lot more vulnerable to heart disease, diabetes, a weakened immune system, sleeplessness, as well as hypertension.

Mental wellness. Chronic anger takes in big quantities of mental power, and also clouds your thinking, making it more challenging to focus or appreciate life. It can additionally bring about anxiety, depression as well as other mental health problems.

Occupation. Constructive criticism, creative differences as well as heated argument can be healthy. However snapping just estranges your colleagues, supervisors, or clients as well as deteriorates their regard.

Relationships. Temper can create enduring scars in the people you love most as well as hinder of relationships and also job relationships. Eruptive anger makes it tough for others to trust you, speak truthfully, or really feel comfortable– as well as is especially damaging to children.

You may really feel like it's out of your hands and also there's little you can do to tame the monster if you have a hot mood. Yet you have a lot more control over your anger than you assume. With understanding regarding the genuine reasons for your temper and also these rage administration tools, you can discover to reveal your emotions without harming others and keep your temper from pirating your life.

Techniques to Tame a Temper: Self-Awareness & Self-Control

Since rage can be effective, handling it is in some cases difficult. It takes lots of self-awareness and also self-discipline to take care of upset feelings. Also, these abilities take time to establish.

Self-awareness is the ability to see what you're assuming as well as really feeling, and also why.

When you get mad, take a moment to observe what you're believing as well as really feeling.

Self-control is everything about believing prior to you acting. It puts some priceless seconds or minutes in between feeling a strong emotion and taking an action you'll be sorry for.

With each other, self-awareness and self-control permit you to have more choice about how to act when you're feeling an extreme feeling like anger.

Preparing to Make a Change

Making a decision to get control of your rage– rather than letting it manage you– means taking a great, difficult look at the ways you've been reacting when you get mad. Struck someone, harmed yourself, or push and also push others around?

For most people who have problem taking advantage of a warm temper, responding similar to this is not what they want. They feel embarrassed by their actions and do not believe it reflects the real them, their ideal selves.

Every person can transform– yet only when they wish to. Believe concerning what you'll acquire from that change, if you desire to make a large change in how you're handling your temper. Even more self-regard? More respect from other individuals? Much less time feeling irritated as well as upset? A more kicked back method to life? Bearing in mind why you wish to make the adjustment can aid.

It can also help to remind yourself that making a change takes time, practice, and patience. Managing anger is about developing new skills and new responses.

How rage monitoring can help you

Many individuals believe that temper monitoring is about finding out to subdue your temper Never getting angry is not a healthy goal. Temper will appear despite how much you attempt to push it down. Truth goal of rage management isn't to suppress feelings of temper, yet instead to recognize the message behind the feeling and reveal it in a healthy means without blowing up. When you do, you'll not only feel much better, you'll additionally be more probable to obtain your demands fulfilled, be better able to take care of dispute in your life, and also enhance your relationships.

Mastering the art of rage monitoring takes job, yet the even more you method, the less complicated it will certainly get. As well as the benefit is massive. Finding how to manage your rage as well as express it appropriately will aid you construct far better relationships, achieve your goals, and also lead a much healthier, more rewarding life.

1: Explore what's actually behind your temper

Have you ever gotten into an argument over something silly? Identifying the real source of frustration will help you communicate your anger better, take constructive action, and work towards a resolution.

Is your anger masking other feelings such as embarrassment, insecurity, hurt, vulnerability, or shame? If your knee-jerk response in many situations is anger, it's likely that your temper is covering up your true feelings.

Anger can also mask anxiety. In the case of the "fight" response, it can often manifest itself as anger or aggression.

Temper issues can come from what you discovered as a child. If you saw others in your family members howl, hit each other, or toss points, you could assume this is just how anger is meant to be expressed.

Temper can be a signs and symptom of another underlying health problem, such as clinical depression, trauma, or chronic stress and anxiety.

Ideas that there's more to your temper than satisfies the eye

You have a tough time compromising.Is it hard for you to understand other individuals' perspectives, as well as even more difficult to yield a point? If you grew up in a family members where temper was out of control, you may bear in mind exactly how the upset person got their method by being the loudest as well as most demanding. Compromising may bring up terrifying sensations of failing and vulnerability.

You see different viewpoints as an individual challenge.Do you think that your method is constantly ideal as well as get angry when others differ? If you have a strong demand to be in control or a fragile vanity, you may analyze various other perspectives as a difficulty to your authority, as opposed to just a different way of taking a look at things.

You have trouble sharing emotions other than anger. Do you satisfaction yourself on being difficult and also in control? Do you really feel that emotions like concern, shame, or shame do not apply to you? Everybody has those emotions so you may be utilizing temper as a cover for them. If you are unpleasant with various emotions, separated, or stuck on a mad one-note reaction to circumstances, it's vital to come back in contact with your sensations. HelpGuide's free Emotional Intelligence Toolkit can assist.

2: Be conscious of your anger warning signs

While you might really feel that you simply blow up into temper without warning, there remain in truth physical indication in your body. Becoming aware of your very own individual indications that your temper is beginning to steam permits you to take actions to manage your anger before it gets out of control.

Take note of the way temper feels in your body:

- Knots in your tummy
- Clinching your hands or jaw
- Feeling clammy or flushed
- Breathing faster
- Frustrations
- Pacing or needing to walk
- " Seeing red"
- Having trouble focusing
- Battering heart

- Tensing your shoulders

3: Identify your triggers

Demanding occasions don't excuse anger, however, understanding how these events impact you can help, you take control of your environment and prevent unneeded irritation. Take a look at your normal routine and attempt to recognize activities, times of day, individuals, places, or situations that activate upset or short-tempered sensations.

Maybe you get involved in a battle whenever you go out for drinks with a specific team of buddies. Or perhaps the web traffic on your everyday commute drives you crazy. When you recognize your triggers, think of methods to either prevent them or see the scenarios in different ways so they don't make your blood boil.

Adverse thought patterns that can trigger rage

You may assume that outside variables– the aloof actions of other people, for instance, or discouraging scenarios– are creating your rage. Temper issues have much less to do with what happens to you than how you translate as well as believe about what took place. Typical negative attitude patterns that fuel and also cause anger include:

Over generalizing. "You ALWAYS interrupt me. You NEVER consider my demands. EVERYBODY disrespects me. I NEVER obtain the credit scores I am worthy of."

Obsessing over "should" as well as "requirements." Having a stiff sight of the means a scenario ought to or have to go and snapping when truth does not line up with this vision.

Telepathic transmission as well as jumping to verdicts. Assuming you "recognize" what another person is really feeling or believing– that they deliberately distress you, ignored your desires, or disrespected you.

Accumulating straws. Seeking things to get distressed about, usually while neglecting or blowing previous anything positive. Allowing these small irritabilities build as well as develop till you reach the "last straw" as well as blow up, frequently over something fairly small.

Criticizing. When anything negative happens or something goes wrong, it's always another person's fault. You tell yourself, "life's not fair," or condemn others for your problems as opposed to taking responsibility for your own life.

When you recognize the thought patterns that sustain your anger, you can discover to reframe exactly how you consider points. Ask yourself: What's the proof that the idea holds true? That it's not real? Is there a much more positive, reasonable way of looking at a circumstance? What would I say to a friend who was thinking these points?

4: Learn ways to cool off swiftly

When you understand just how to identify the indication that your temper is increasing as well as anticipate your triggers, you can act quickly to take care of your temper prior to it draws out of control. There are many techniques that can help you cool off as well as keep your anger in check.

Concentrate on the physical feelings of anger. While it may appear counterproductive, adjusting into the means your body really feels when you're upset usually lessens the emotional strength of your anger.

Take some deep breaths. Deep, sluggish breathing helps combat increasing tension. The trick is to breathe deeply from the abdominal area, obtaining as much fresh air as feasible right into your lungs.

Get moving. A brisk walk around the block is a great concept. Exercise launches pent-up power so you can come close to the circumstance with a cooler head.

Use your senses. You can make use of view, scent, touch, hearing, as well as preference to quickly soothe stress and anxiety and cool off. You could attempt paying attention to a favored composition, looking at a cherished picture, appreciating a favorite, or rubbing a pet dog.

Stretch or massage therapy locations of tension. Roll your shoulders if you are tensing them, for instance, or carefully massage therapy your neck and scalp.

Slowly countto ten. Focus on the counting to allow your logical mind to catch up with your feelings. Start counting once more if you still really feel out of control by the time you reach ten.

Offer yourself a truth check.

Take a minute to believe regarding the situation when you begin getting upset about something. Ask yourself:

- Exactly how essential is it in the grand plan of things?
- Is it really worth getting angry about it?
- Is it worth destroying the rest of my day?

- Is my action appropriate to the circumstance?
- Is there anything I can do concerning it?
- Is taking action worth my time?

5: Find healthier ways to share your temper

If you've determined that the situation deserves getting angry regarding and also there's something you can do to make it much better, the key is to share your feelings in a healthy means. Knowing just how to fix dispute in a positive method will certainly assist you enhance your relationships rather than harming them.

Constantly fight fair. It's okay to be distressed at someone, yet if you don't fight fair, the relationship will rapidly break down. Fighting fair allows you to share your very own needs while still appreciating others.

Make the partnership your priority. Maintaining as well as strengthening the partnership, rather than "winning" the debate, should constantly be your initial concern. Regard the various other individual and their viewpoint.

Concentrate on the present. It's easy to start tossing previous grievances right into the mix when you are in the warmth of suggesting. Instead of focusing to the past as well as assigning blame, focus on what you can do in the here and now to resolve the issue.

Agree to forgive. If you're unable or resistant to forgive, Resolving conflict is difficult. Resolution lies in releasing the urge to punish, which can never compensate for our losses and only contributes to our injury by additional depleting as well as draining our lives.

If thingsget too heated, take five. Remove yourself from the circumstance for a few minutes or for as lengthy as it takes you to cool down if your rage starts to spiral out of control.

Know when to let something go. It takes 2 individuals to keep an argument going.

6: Stay calm by taking care of yourself

Taking care of your overall mental and also physical wellbeing can help to relieve tension as well as occasional rage issues.

Manage tension. If your tension levels are with the high, you're more likely to have a hard time regulating your temper. Attempt practicing leisure strategies such as mindfulness reflection, modern muscle mass leisure, or deep breathing. You'll really feel calmer as well as much more in control of your feelings.

Chatting about your feelings and seeking a different perspective on a situation is not the exact same as venting. Merely venting your temper at a person will only fuel your temper and also reinforce your rage problem.

Get enough rest. A lack of rest can exacerbate adverse ideas and also leave you feeling flustered as well as short-fused. Try to obtain seven to nine hours of good quality sleep.

Exercise on a regular basis. It's an efficient way to burn-off stress and also simplicity stress and anxiety, and also it can leave you feeling much more relaxed as well as positive throughout the day. Aim for at the very least 30 mins on the majority of days, separated into shorter durations if that's much easier.

Be clever concerning alcohol as well as medications. They reduced your restraints as well as can make it also harder to manage your rage. Also consuming too much caffeine can make you extra cranky and vulnerable to rage.

7: Use wit to relieve stress

When points get stressful, humor and also playfulness can assist you lighten the mood, smooth over distinctions, reframe issues, and keep things in viewpoint. Attempt utilizing a little laid-back wit when you feel yourself getting upset in a situation. It can allow you to get your point throughout without getting the various other person's defenses up or harming their sensations.

Prevent mockery, mean-spirited wit. If in doubt, begin by utilizing self-deprecating wit. If you've made a blunder at job or you've simply spilled coffee over yourself, instead of getting upset or selecting a battle, attempt making a joke about it.

When wit and also play are made use of to lower tension as well as anger, a potential dispute can even become a chance for better connection and affection.

8: Recognize if you need professional assistance

If, in spite of placing these previous rage administration strategies right into technique, your anger is still spiraling out of hand, or if you're getting into problem with the regulation or harming others, you need more assistance.

Anger administration courses allow you to satisfy others managing the exact same battles and find out pointers and methods for managing your temper.

Therapy, either team or individual, can be a wonderful way to check out the factors behind your anger and also identify triggers. Therapy can additionally provide a refuge to practice new skills for sharing anger.

Anger isn't the real issue in a violent connection

In spite of what many think, domestic physical violence and also abuse does not take place because of the abuser's loss of control over their mood. Rather, it's a deliberate option to control an additional person. If you are abusive towards your spouse or partner, recognize that you require customized treatment, not routine rage administration courses.

Communication skills

Communication issues can raise any family's stress level. When a family member has co-occurring conditions, communications can, in some cases, call for additional effort. Mental health disorders can create individuals to withdraw or misinterpret individuals or miss social signs. Compound use can better complicate interactions by worsening psychiatric signs or driving dishonest and disruptive actions.

Effective interaction serves as precautionary maintenance, reassuring relative that they respect each other as well as value each other's initiatives. Great day-to-day communication can additionally make it much easier to bring up concerns, make requests when needed, as well as settle conflict when it arises.

How Can Co-occurring Disorders Affect Communication in a Family?

When a relative has co-occurring problems, communication might take additional effort and recognition on everyone's part. Sometimes a psychiatric condition can impede a person's communication. The person may

- take out and not talk when feeling depressed
- feel irritable, have mad outbursts, or act unpredictably as a result of mood instability
- perceive other individuals inaccurately, which can cause social anxiousness or paranoia
- make unreasonable demands of others, or reveal an absence of concern for them, as a result of preoccupation with concerns or anxiety

- miss out on or misinterpret usual social cues, such as facial expressions or tips, which can result in misconceptions

When the individual likewise has a material use condition, these troubles can be multiplied:

Communications with others can be influenced by the instant impacts important use, yearnings, or withdrawal signs.

Addiction-related conflicts with others can develop, arising from lies, broken promises, or failure to fulfill responsibilities.

Material use can aggravate the signs and symptoms of psychiatric disorders as well as disrupt adhering to therapy suggestions.

Excellent interactions can aid resolve conflict in an effective method, let member of the family be listened to, and also help them remain linked to each other. Home group work can help homes work on important interaction abilities, and also the handout "Effective Communication" from the Co-occurring Disorders Program supplies a variety of methods for relative. Here is an excerpt:

Specify

Be quick and also up-front when you're talking with someone with co-occurring disorders. Wordy, ambiguous declarations are hard for anyone to follow, however, specifically somebody that has difficulty concentrating-as do many people with psychological wellness conditions and/or substance use problems. Specify rapidly to ensure you are listened to as well as recognized.

Express Feelings Clearly with "I" Statements

Explain your very own sensations and also stay clear of putting others on the defensive. By utilizing words such as "angry," "happy," "upset," or "worried," you can inform your own fact as well as help protect against the misunderstandings that can occur when people have to think each other's sensations.

" I" statements, such as "I really feel anxious when ...," are direct, as well as they make an impression. When distressed sensations are involved, "I" statements work better than criticizing "you" statements. Instead of saying, "You pissed me off when you were late for dinner last evening" (a condemning declaration), try this: "I was upset when you came home late for supper last night. I would certainly appreciate it if you 'd be on time or call if you're going to be late."

Promote Yourself as well as Not for Others

Due to the fact that they think they know what the various other individual is feeling, individuals typically speak for others. In some homes this takes the form of indirect "backchannel interaction" (for instance, "Your mommy is angry with you"). Be alert to these habits and attempt to transform them.

All of these habits naturally lead to misunderstandings-since each person is truly an expert on only his or her feelings – this may seem hard at first for family members who are not used to direct communication.

Focus on Behaviors Rather Than on Traits

People can alter their behavior-what they do-more conveniently than they can transform interior qualities or traits such as personality, mindsets, or sensations. When you are distressed with somebody's activities, concentrate your communication on behavior as opposed to on qualities, making it clear what you are dismayed about. Make it a total statement, linked to habits.

For example:

As opposed to saying: "I'm worried regarding your health and wellness."

Say: "I'm worried regarding your wellness since you've begun consuming alcohol once again."

Instead of stating: "You're thoughtless due to the fact that you only think of yourself."

Claim: "I occasionally believe you do not care about me because you seldom ask about my feelings. I wish you would certainly reveal a lot more concern by asking how I'm feeling more frequently."

Impulse control

An individual with an impulse control disorder is usually incapable to withstand the sudden, forceful impulse to do something that may go against the legal rights of others or produce conflict with social norms. These spontaneous behaviors may occur repeatedly, promptly and also without factor to consider of the consequences of that actions. Pyromania (intentionally starting fires) and also kleptomania (the urge to steal) are popular instances, but there are others.

Signs and Symptoms

There are some signs and symptoms that might point to an impulse control condition in some people. It is not always simple to identify a condition, but the complying with flags may be create for attention.

Behavioral signs and symptoms: For example, stealing, lying, starting fires, risky or promiscuous actions, as well as hostile or unpredictable habits.

Cognitive signs: Obsessive behavior, being short-tempered or agitated, flying into a rage, and poor focus abilities, to name a few.

Social and psychological symptoms that frequently show up as reduced self-esteem, being socially withdrawn or separated, seeming removed and/or nervous, experiencing radical shifts in thoughts and also moods, and having sensations of guilt or remorse.

When a Behavior Becomes a Disorder

Commonly, the impulsive activity results from tension that has developed to the point where the person can no more resist it. The prompt feeling of remedy for acting upon the spontaneous actions is just short-term, nevertheless.

Sensations such as guilt or shame may follow, and also repeated spontaneous acts may bring about a variety of unfavorable repercussions, such as better psychological distress or regret, in the long-lasting.

When the emotional toll or impulsive actions becomes unrestrainable or seriously interrupts daily life, an impulse control problem is a likely reason.

Danger Factors

Both external and also internal stress factors are understood triggers for damaged control. Numerous sorts of impulse control problems are thought to originate from underlying neurological vulnerabilities paired with environmental stress and anxieties.

Some risk aspects consist of:

- Being male (Males are extra susceptible to impulse control problems than women).
- Hereditary proneness.
- Chronic drug or alcohol use.
- Undergoing misuse, overlook, or trauma.
- Direct exposure to violence or aggressiveness.

Certain sorts of "chemical imbalances" may contribute to an impulse control disorder in some people. Additional mental wellness problems, such as depression or obsessive-compulsive disorder (OCD), commonly exist together in people with an impulse control condition.

Common Types and also Treatments.

The term impulse control problem is presently a group of psychological health issue that consist of disruptive, impulse-control, and perform problems.

Some typical kinds of impulse control conditions consist of:

Pyromania

Individuals with this impulse control disorder purposely begin fires without regard to the devastation or injury their activities might trigger. It prevails for many convicted arsonists with apparent pyromania to also have personality disorders such as borderline as well as antisocial personality disorders.

Treatment of this impulse disorder often includes addressing any underlying mental disease pharmacologically. Cognitive behavior modification strategies have also been used.

Intermittent Explosive Disorder

Intermittent explosive disorderis detected when an individual has, on several celebrations, acted upon hostile impulses and dedicated seriously hostile acts, such as assault or destruction of building. One way it's identified is by the severity of the individual's hostile behavior (it's well out of proportion to the trigger that preceded it).

Research studies have located a web link between the experience of a terrible occasion and also intermittent explosive disorder.

Individuals with the intermittent explosive disordermay benefit from treatment that consists of both medicine as well as cognitive behavior modification.

Kleptomania

This is the continuous and tempting urge to steal. Kleptomania is unusual in that, unlike more common burglars, an individual with this impulse control problem might usually steal things that have little personal or financial value.

Kleptomania may have subtypes that are more like obsessive-compulsive disorder (OCD), and others that are more similar to addictive and also mood conditions. It prevails for people with kleptomania (as well as their first-degree family members) to have various other comorbid psychological or addiction problems.

Reliable treatment options for kleptomania may vary depending upon the subtype noticeable in the person. Cognitive behavior therapy and medication have been shown to be effective. Lithium, anti-epileptics, as well as opioid antagonist medicines have actually revealed promise in specific situations.

Problem-solving skills

Have you ever before thought about yourself as a trouble solver? I'm guessing not. In truth, we are continuously fixing troubles. Also the far better our problem resolving abilities are, the simpler our lives are.

Problems arise in many forms and forms. They can be mundane, everyday troubles, or bigger more complicated issues:

- What to have for supper tonight?
- Which path to take to function?
- Just how to fix a project that's running behind schedule?

Just how to change from an unexciting job to a job you're actually enthusiastic about?

On a daily basis, you'll be confronted with at the very least one trouble to address. Yet it gets much easier when you recognize that problems are merely choices. There's absolutely nothing "scary" regarding them aside from having to decide.

No matter what job you're in, where you live, who your companion is, the number of friends you have, you will be judged on your ability to address problems. Due to the fact that problems equivalent headaches for every person worried as well as individuals don't know of such trouble. The extra troubles you can fix, the less inconvenience; overall, the happier people are with you. Everyone wins.

Why Are Problem Solving Skills Important?

Issue is something tough to understand or accomplish or deal with. It can be a task, a situation, or perhaps an individual. Problem solving involves methods and abilities to locate the very best remedies to problems.

Problem resolving is very important because all of us have decisions to make, as well as inquiries to answer in our lives. Incredible people like Eleanor

Roosevelt, Steve Jobs, Mahatma Gandhi as well as Martin Luther King Jr., are all wonderful issues solvers. Good parents, instructors, medical professionals and stewards all have to be good at addressing various kind of troubles also.

Problem addressing skills are for our daily lives.

Exactly How to Enhance Problem Solving Skills

Many people think that you need to be very smart in order to be a good problem solver, but that's not true.

You do not need to be extremely smart to be an problem solver, you simply require technique.

When you comprehend the various actions to resolve a trouble, you'll be able to generate great options.

1. Focus on the Solution, Not the Problem

Neuroscientists have shown that your mind can not discover solutions if you focus on the issue. This is since when you concentrate on the trouble, you're successfully feeding "negativity," which in turn triggers negative emotions in the mind.

I'm not saying you ought to "neglect the problem," instead, try to remain calm. It aids to first, acknowledge the issue; and after that, relocate your focus to a solution-oriented attitude where you maintain chosen what the "response" could be, instead of sticking around on "what went wrong" and also "that's mistake it is."

"2. Adapt "5 Whys" to Clearly Define the Problem

"5 Whys" is a problem addressing framework to aid you reach the origin of a problem.

By repetitively asking the concern "why" on a problem, you can explore the root cause of a problem, and that's exactly how you can find the most effective remedy to deal with the root issue finally. Also, it can go deeper than simply asking why for five times.

For instance, If the problem is "always late to work:"

Why am I late to work?

I constantly click the snooze switch and also simply want to take place resting.

Why do I intend to go on sleeping?

I feel so exhausted in the morning.

Why do I feel exhausted in the early morning?

I rested late the evening before, that's why.

Why did I sleep late?

I wasn't drowsy after consuming coffee, as well as I simply maintained scrolling my Facebook feed as well as somehow I could not stop.

Why did I drink coffee?

Not having sufficient sleep the night before since I was also drowsy at work in the mid-day.

So there you see, if you really did not try to dig out the root of the issue, you may just set a couple of more alarm systems as well as have it beep every 5 minutes in the morning. In fact, the problem you require to solve is to give up Facebook browsing constantly at evening so you'll really feel a lot more energetic in the day time, and you will not also require coffee.

3. Streamline Things

As people, we tend to make things much more challenging than they require to be! Try simplifying your issue by generalizing it.

Remove all the details as well as return to the basics. Try looking for an actually simple, apparent service– you might be amazed at the outcomes! As well as all of us know that it's often the easy things that are one of the most effective.

4. Note out as Many Solutions as Possible

Attempt to come up with "ALL POSSIBLE SOLUTIONS"– even if they seem ludicrous at. It's essential you keep an open mind to improve creativity, which can trigger prospective remedies.

Originating from 10 years in the corporate advertising and marketing sector, it is drummed into you that "No idea is a bad idea," and also this help creative thinking in brainstorms as well as other analytic methods.

Whatever you do, do not ridicule yourself for thinking of "foolish solutions" as it's typically the crazy concepts that cause other much more viable services.

5. Believe Laterally

Adjustment the 'direction' of your thoughts by assuming laterally. Pay attention to the saying,

"You cannot dig an opening in a various areasby excavating it deeper."

Attempt to transform your method and also take a look at points in a new way. You can attempt flipping your purpose around and trying to find a remedy that is the polar contrary!

Even if it really feels silly, a special and fresh method typically promotes a fresh solution.

6. Use Language That Creates Possibility

Lead your reasoning with phrases like "suppose ..." and
"visualize if ..." These terms open up our minds to assume artistically as well as encourage remedies.

Stay clear of closed, unfavorable language such as 'I don't assume ...' or 'But this is not right ...'.

There's nothing terrifying concerning an issue when you begin to adapt my recommendations.

Attempt not to see issues as "scary" points! If you consider what an issue truly is, it's truly simply comments on your present circumstance.

Every problem is informing you that something is not currently working which you need to find a new method around it.

Try to plan problems neutrally– without any type of judgment. Practice focusing on specifying an issue, keep one's cool and also not to make things too made complex.

FAMILY THERAPY

A psycho therapist will certainly deal with the whole family members to make changes. This can aid parents find support and also learn techniques for handling their child's ODD.

What is Family Therapy/ Family Counseling?

Family members treatment or family members counseling is a type of treatment that is developed to resolve particular problems influencing the health and wellness and also performance of a family. It can be utilized to aid a family members through a difficult period, a major transition, or mental or behavioral health issue in family members.

As Dr. Michael Herkov explains, family members therapy views people' issues in the context of the larger device: the family members. The presumption of this type of treatment is that troubles cannot be successfully addressed or resolved without understanding the characteristics of the group.

The way the family operates influences just how the customer's issues created and just how they are encouraged or allowed by other participants of their home.

Home treatment can use techniques and workouts from cognitive therapy, behavior modification, social therapy, or various other kinds of individual therapy. Like with various other kinds of treatment, the methods used will certainly depend on the specific issues the customer or customers present with.

Emotional or behavioral troubles in children are common reasons to visit a family members therapist. A child's troubles do not exist in a vacuum; they exist, and will likely require to be addressed, within the context of the family members.

It should be noted that in family treatment or therapy, the term "family members" does not necessarily suggest blood relatives. In this context, "family" is any individual who "plays a long-lasting helpful function in one's life, which might not mean blood relations or family members in the exact same home."

According to Licensed Clinical Social Worker Laney Cline King, these are the most typical kinds of family treatment:

Bowenian: This form of home treatment is finest fit for circumstances in which people cannot or do not want to involve other member of the family in the treatment. Bowenian treatment is built on two core ideas: triangulation (the natural tendency to vent or distress by talking with a third party) and differentiation (learning to come to be less emotionally reactive in family relationships);

Structural: Structural treatment focuses on reinforcing the family and adjusting system to ensure that the parents remain in control and that both adults and also children set appropriate borders. In this form of treatment, the therapist "joins" the family members in order to observe, learn, as well as boost their capability to aid the home strengthen their partnerships;

Systemic: The Systemic model refers to the kind of therapy that concentrates on the unconscious interactions as well as definitions behind relative' habits. The specialist in this type of treatment is neutral and also distant, enabling the family members to dive deeper into their concerns and issues as a family;

Strategic: This type of therapy is straighter and also shorter than the others, in which the therapist assigns homework to the family. This research is planned to alter the means member of the family interact by examining as well as changing the method the family interacts and chooses. The specialist takes the position of power in this sort of treatment, which permits other family members who might not usually hold as much power to connect better.

What is a Family Counselor Trained For?

As the various kinds of therapy explained above program, a family specialist might be hired to tackle many different functions. These many functions require a home specialist to go through a lot of training, formal education, as well as screening to ensure that the specialist is up to the job.

" In this therapy, the specialist takes duty for the outcome of the treatment. This has nothing to do with bad or great, sense of guilt or virtue, right or incorrect. It is the straightforward acknowledgement that you make a difference."– Eileen Bobrow.

While specialists might have various approaches and also preferred therapy strategies, they have to all contend least a minimum degree of experience with the therapy of:

- Child as well as adolescent behavioral issues;

- Grieving;

- Depression and anxiety;

- LGBTQ concerns;

- Domestic violence;

- Infertility;

- Marital disputes;

Chemical abuse.

In order to deal with these as well as various other family members issues, therapists must:

- Observe just how people communicate within groups;

- Resolve as well as evaluate connection troubles;

- Diagnose as well as deal with psychological disorders within a home context;

- Guide customers via transitional dilemmas such as separation or fatality;

- Highlight bothersome relational or behavior patterns;

- Help change inefficient actions with healthy and balanced choices; and

- Take an alternative (mind-body) strategy to health.

What is the Goal of Family Therapy?

" To put the globe right in order, we must initially put the nation in order; to place the country in order, we must initially put the family in order; to place the home in order, we need to first grow our individual life; we should initially set our hearts right."– Confucius.

In short, the goal of home treatment is to interact to heal any mental, psychological, or emotional issues tearing your family apart. What is the goal of family therapy?To guide a family members towards a healthy and balanced life, family members specialists intend to help individuals in improving communication, addressing family issues, comprehending and taking care of family members situations, and producing a far better home atmosphere.

The goals of home treatment depend on the here and now issues of the clients. For instance, goals may differ based upon the complying with circumstances.

A family member is struggling with schizophrenia or severe psychosis: The objective is to assist other relative understand the disorder and get used to the mental adjustments that the client might be undergoing.

Issues emerging from cross-generational boundaries, such as when parents share a home with grandparents, or children are being raised by grandparents: The objective is to boost interaction and help the member of the family set healthy borders.

Families differing social standards (single parents, gay pairs raising children, etc.): The objectives below are not always to resolve any kind of particular interior troubles, however the member of the family may require aid dealing external factors like social mindsets.

Family members who originate from combined racial, social, or spiritual histories: The goal is to aid member of the family additionally their understanding of each other and also develop healthy and balanced connections.

One member is being scapegoated or having their treatment in private therapy undermined: When one family member is battling with feeling like the outcast or obtains limited assistance from various other family members, the goal is to facilitate raised compassion and also understanding for the individual within their family members and provide assistance for them to proceed their treatment.

The person's problems appear completely connected to troubles with other relative: In cases where the issue or issues are deeply rooted in problems with other relative, the objective is to resolve each of the contributing issues and also address or reduce the results of this pattern of troubles.

A blended family members (i.e., step-family): Blended families can struggle with problems special to their situations. In combined families, the goal of home treatment is to improve understanding as well as assist in healthy and balanced interactions between family members.

What are the Benefits of Family Therapy?

This more holistic strategy to treating troubles within a family members has verified to be very effective in many cases. In home treatment, family members can work on their troubles with the assistance of a mental wellness expert in a regulated as well as risk-free setting.

The benefits of family treatment consist of:

- A much better understanding of healthy borders as well as family members patterns as well as dynamics

- Enhanced interaction

- Improved problem solving

- Deeper empathy

Decreased problem and also better rage monitoring skills.More particularly, home treatment can enhance family relationships via:

- Bringing the family members together after a crisis

- Creating sincerity between member of the family

- Instilling rely on member of the family

- Developing an encouraging family atmosphere

- Reducing sources of tension and also anxiety within the family

- Helping relative forgive each other

- Conflict resolution for family members

Restoring relative that have been isolated.

Family members therapy enhances the skills needed for healthy home functioning, including interaction, problem resolution, and analytical. Improving these skills additionally boosts the potential for success in resolving and getting rid of family problems.

In home therapy, the focus is on supplying all family members with the tools they need to promote healing.

Examples and Exercises

If family members therapy seems like a treatment that would certainly profit you and also your loved ones, the best course of action is to find a qualified specialist with whom you can construct an excellent working partnership and address the troubles your family members is dealing with.

Nevertheless, if you're not quite ready for this action, or there are obstacles in between you and obtaining treatment, there are many workouts as well as suggestions that you might discover to be good choices.

The exercises and techniques below are suggested to be utilized within the context of a healing working relationship, yet some additionally have applications for those that desire to check out the possibilities of family therapy prior to dedicating to long-lasting therapy with a specialist. You may find these workouts to be useful enhancements to your treatment toolbox if you are a specialist or various other mental health professional.

The Miracle Question

This exercise can be used in specific, pairs, or home therapy, and also is meant to help the customer(s) explore the type of future they would like to construct. Most of us struggle sometimes, however sometimes the struggle is better because we merely do not know what our objectives actually are.

The Miracle Question is an exceptional method to help the client or customers probe their own dreams as well as needs. When used in the context of couples or family members treatment, it can assist customers in understanding what their significant other or member of the family needs in order to be happy with their partnership.

This Miracle Question is posed as complies with:

" Suppose this evening, while you slept, a miracle happened. When you awake tomorrow, what would be a few of things you would certainly see that would certainly inform your life had instantly improved?"

While the client may provide a response that is an unfeasibility in their waking life, their response can still serve. If they do provide an impossible solution, the therapist can dive deeper right into the clients' favored miracle with this inquiry: "How would certainly that make a distinction?"

This question aids both the specialist and also the customer– the client in imagining a positive future in which their troubles are attended to or mitigated, and also the specialist in learning just how they can best help their client in their sessions.

Colored Candy Go Around

If you're searching for a fun as well as creative icebreaker or introduction to family treatment, this exercise can be a great way to start.

To take part in this exercise with your family, you require a bundle of Skittles, M&M s, or a similar colorful candy. Distribute seven items to every relative, and also advise them to arrange their sweet by shade (and refraining from eating it just yet!).

Next, ask a member of the family to select a shade and also share how many they have. For nonetheless many candies of this color they have, advise them to provide the same variety of actions to the following motivates based on the color:

- Green– words to describe your family;

- Purple– ways your family has fun;

- Orange–things you wish to boost regarding your family;

- Red–things you stress over;

- Yellow– preferred memories with your home.

Colored Candy Go Around family therapy tools

When the very first member of the family has actually offered their responses, tell them to select the following member of the family to address the exact same timely based upon the number of candies that person has.

As soon as the question has been answered, the sweets can be eaten.

When all family members have replied to these prompts, launch a conversation based upon the solutions supplied by the home. The complying with inquiries can promote discussion:

What did you discover?

What was one of the most unusual thing you learnt more about somebody else?

Exactly how will you function towards making changes/improvements?

Other thanthe high sugar content in this exercise, you can see that this is a wonderful game to have fun with children! If this seems like a valuable exercise that you wish to attempt with your family members, you can discover more information and also directions on page 3 of this PDF from specialist Liana Lowenstein.

Emotions Ball

This is a straightforward exercise, calling for only a round and a pen or pen to create with. It is frequently utilized with children and teenagers in many contexts, as it takes the stress off of speaking about feelings, for those that may be uncomfortable sharing them.

A coastline ball is an ideal ball for this activity– big sufficient to create several emotions on and very easy to throw back as well as forth in a circle. Write several feelings on the ball, such as "joyous," "lonesome," "silly," or "sad."

Collect your family members into a circle as well as start to toss the round to and fro in between family members. When a relative captures the sphere, have them define a time when they felt the emotion facing them. You might have the catcher act out a feeling, a task specifically fit for children.

The intent of this workout is to talk about feelings with your family members and method listening to one another and also sharing your sensations.

The Family Gift.

This workout can help a specialist to learn more about a family much better. If you are using it without the assistance of a therapist, it can aid you to further your understanding of your very own family members as well as provoke thoughtful discussion.

Clarify to the family that they are going to produce a present from the products supplied. They should make a decision together on this gift as well as how it can be utilized within their home.

They have 30 minutes to pick this gift and craft it. Once they have developed the present, they have to put it in the gift bag. Within the context of family members treatment, this workout offers the therapist with an understanding of the inner workings of the home, how they make decisions as well as overall work as a unit.

If you are taking part in this workout as a home without the presence of a specialist, it can aid you to begin a meaningful discussion.

Use these questions or prompts to promote the conversation:

- Describe your present.
- Tell just how you each felt as you were producing your present.
- Who made the decisions? Who determined what the gift should be?
- Were two or more individuals in your home able to function well with each other?
- Did anybody trigger any kind of difficulties or differences, as well as if so, just how was this dealt with?
- Is anything regarding the way you did the task that advises you of exactly how things operate in your family members in the house?
- Exactly how can the gift aid your family members? What else can assist your family?

There is a wide range of information to be gained from observing these kinds of communications or engaging in these kinds of discussion.

Mirroring Activity.

This enjoyable workout is a fantastic method to aid member of the family relate to each other and also collaborate.

The activity can be clarified to a family members by the therapist with the complying with instructions:

"I desire you to stand in front of me just right there (pointing to a place about two feet before the professional). You are going to be my mirror. Everything I do you will certainly attempt to copy, but the technique is to replicate me at exactly the exact same time that I am doing it, to make sure that you are my mirror. I will certainly go gradually so you have a possibility to think of where I will certainly be moving; therefore, we can do it exactly at the same time. We cannot touch each other. I will lead first and then you will certainly follow. Ready? Here we go!".

Matching video game family treatment.

First, the therapist can design this workout with among the relative, then that individual can take a turn leading another.

This is an especially valuable exercise for children, but it can be used with relative of any age. It requires the family members to provide each other their full attention, cooperate with one another, and also communicate with both words and also body language.

It also enables the member of the family to become extra in tune with each other and can be used with brother or sisters, a parent, a child, and even couples in marriage counseling.

Genogram

A genogram is a graphic or schematic depiction of a client's family tree. Nevertheless, unlike the regular family history, the genogram provides far more info on the relationships among family members.

It can be utilized to draw up blood relations, medical conditions in the family, and also, frequently in the case of family therapy, emotional connections.

Genograms consist of two (2) levels of information– that which exists on the standard family history which provides a lot more detailed check out the home:

Fundamental Information: name, gender, day of birth, date of fatality (if any kind of).

Extra Information: education, line of work, major life events, persistent diseases, social behaviors, nature of family relationships, emotional partnerships, social partnerships, alcohol addiction, depression, diseases, partnerships, as well as living situations.

By including this additional info, the specialist and also client can interact to determine patterns in the family background that may have influenced the customer's existing emotions and actions. Occasionally the basic act of mapping out and also observing this info can explain things that were formerly unnoticed.

The information on psychological connections can consist of points of interest and also any kind of facets of the relationship that may have impacted the client(s), such as whether the partnership is marked by abuse, whether a marital relationship is divided or undamaged, if a relationship is defined by love or indifference, whether a relationship could be thought about "regular" or dysfunctional. This workout could be completed independently, yet it is most likely to be most efficient when finished combined with a certified specialist.

Other treatment

peer groups: The child can discover exactly how to boost their social abilities as well as relationships with other children.

Medications: These can aid deal with root causes of ODD, such as clinical depression or ADHD. Nevertheless, there is no specific drug to treat ODD itself.

Therapy– Children find out how to share and also control their anger. It might be alone, with family members, or in a support system. Many types may be used.

Social abilities training– Helps your child deal with and also control disappointment with their peers.

FIVE TRAITS OF A STRONG PARENT

Being a successful parent supports establish high qualities in children such as honesty, empathy, self-discipline, self-direction, participation, happiness and compassion, and imparts in them the inspiration to attain, according to writer as well as Temple University psychology teacher Laurence Steinberg. The function of a great parent is also to shield their child from creating emotional troubles, such as clinical depression, anxiousness as well as anti-social habits, which boosts the risk of substance misuse.

Loving and Affectionate

A research of 2,000 parents performed by psychology professor and scientist Robert Epstein, that was published in a 2010 issue of "Scientific American," found that being loving and also affectionate while still providing parental guidance was most vital in raising happy children. Loving parents choose to respect, motivate and also support their children rather than judging and condemning them. A loving parent could say, "It's great that you cleaned your space without being asked" or "I'm so honored that you made the basketball group."

Skilled Communicators

Parents who are skillful communicators reveal real rate of interest in all areas of their child's life and are constantly readily available for him. To end up being a competent communicator, encourage your child to express his feelings and then pay attention with understanding.

Capacity to Manage Stress

One more important quality of a good parent is the capacity to handle their stress as well as temper, which leads to well-adjusted children, according to Epstein. Children commonly handle stress and anxiety by mirroring how their parents manage emotions throughout difficult situations.

Respectful of Autonomy

Disobedience on celebration is a healthy and balanced component of your child's attempt to develop his freedom. Instead of determining guidelines, they ask for their child's input as well as make establishing guidelines a shared job. Children that are allowed to take part in making choices end up being a lot more determined to carry them out, according to the Children Health web site.

Favorable Role Model

Being a positive good example for appropriate behavior is more reliable than specific corrective measures or training in increasing your children, according to a 2010 article at PsychologyToday.com. Children learn through observation as well as usually imitate the behavior of their parents. When they see their parents saying as well as losing control, they really feel less secure. They could attempt to settle disputes by saying and also dealing with, just like their parents do. Yet parents that are able to work out their disputes and also disputes via tranquil discussions rather than heated debates come to be healthy and balanced role models. Be those qualities you want to develop in your child, such as generosity, empathy, honesty, respectfulness, resistance, persistence, honesty as well as genuine love.

QUALITIES TO NURTURE IN YOUR CHILD

Professionals state that effective, happy individuals– those that succeed in their picked careers and develop satisfying relationships throughout their lives– have a tendency to share specific top qualities. As well as parents can assist support those vital traits in their children, even when they're babies. Here's a look at the top five qualities your baby will certainly need, according to child-development specialists, together with some means you can start your child on the path to getting each of these necessary assets.

1. Depend on

A fundamental count on others is the structure on which all other traits remainder. Without this particular, babies encounter an uphill developmental battle.

She'll have a hard time building relationships, feeling great, and moving on unless she has the capacity to depend on, says Debbie Phillips, a child-development expert with Work/Family Directions, a consulting firm in Boston.

Presenting depend on starts right from the time your infant is birthed. You can bond with your baby in a manner that instills in her a profound complacency, a confidence worldwide– and eventually, in herself. In infancy, that indicates responding to her fundamental demands. Feed her when she's starving. Rock her with she wants to be cuddled, alter her diaper when it's dirtied. Likewise make the most of your day-to-day communications by talking to her, singing to her, and also making eye contact touch with. To produce an actually safe feeling, introduce rituals such as checking out a tale every night before bedtime.

Your child's needs come to be extra intricate when she's a young child. Certainly she needs to be fed, bathed, and looked after, however she also needs you to look at her scribbles and also her block towers. Acknowledging her achievements may not seem as vital as, say, giving her supper, however it is. She'll tell you in her own method, "I need you to discover this," states Susan Landry, PhD, a developmental psychotherapist at the University of Texas Medical School in Houston. Attempt to pay attention to her signals and also react appropriately to her requirements.

Not all children are alike and your little one will trust you a lot more if you customize your activities to suit her personality. The more you reveal your infant you comprehend her specific personality, the more she'll feel that you're on her side.

2. Patience

It's real: Good things come to those that wait. Children that learn persistence have the ability to persist and are more probable to do well, claims Claire Lerner, a child-development expert with Zero to Three, an advocacy group that focuses on toddlers and also infants. Instructing a child the top quality of patience can aid infuse in him a sensation of freedom and also achievement.

Intend to help your child along? Remember this: Your child is experiencing. If you fly off the handle when you meet harsh traffic or a lengthy line, you'll establish a bad instance. They're like sponges, taking whatever in, says Jody Johnston Pawel, a parent teacher and writer of The Parent's Tool shop: The Universal Blueprint for Building a Healthy Family. Specialists call it modeling– do the ideal point and your child is more probable to follow. Become rapidly irritated when your young child splashes his milk as well as you'll share one message; smoothly aid him clean it up and also, you'll teach him something else completely.

Connecting words to your little one's emotions additionally aids foster persistence. Toddlers normally cannot talk a whole lot, but they recognize many of what you inform them.

Young children don't have the exact same feeling of time that we do, which makes it also harder for them to be understood. You can assist by marking time in methods besides minutes as well as hours. As an example, if your child requests some juice when you're in the center of washing , instead of responding with, "I'll get it in five mins," try saying

"I'll get it as quickly as I'm finished with these plates." This way, he can watch your development and evaluate exactly how soon he'll get his juice.

3. Responsibility

To succeed in life, says Doreen Virtue, PhD, a psychotherapist in Los Angeles and author of Your Emotions, Yourself, you need to know how to follow through commitments you make. It's something that even a baby can begin to tackle.

Specifically, that implies you can start thinking about child-sized obligations, like handing her a spoon as well as asking her to give it to Dad. As she gets older, you can make duties advanced, perhaps asking her to throw her socks in the hamper with or pile her books. If you also explain the value of each task, you'll make it all that much more palatable. Make sure to keep your explanations brief to avoid confusion; for example, the hamper is "where dirty clothes go to get clean," and stacking books "makes it easy to find what you want to read next time." She might not comprehend your descriptions initially, but ultimately the ideas will sink in.

Helping to clean is, of course, a useful chore. Try making it a game or singing a special clean-up song while you put the toys away.

Naturally, we're usually so hurried that we inhibit our children from doing tasks due to the fact that it takes them also long. Choose one or two key responsibilities– but make sure you enforce them if you're pressed for time.

4. Compassion

Empathy is crucial to the development of an individual's social proficiency, states Phillips. To have successful connections, you have to know exactly how people are really feeling as well as respond suitably. While also infants show a primitive type of compassion, children do not really end up being with the ability of putting themselves in someone's shoes up until someplace between the ages of 3 as well as 6. Prior to then, they have trouble seeing the world from any person's point of view but their own. When a 2-year-old bops his close friend on the head, he doesn't understand that it hurts because he hasn't felt anything himself, says Phillips.

There's a lot you can do to help a child develop empathy. If you see another child with a skinned knee, talk about how it must sting. This is one quality that needs a lot of repeating before you can expect it to take, says Pawel.

A 1998 study done at Yale University showed that preschoolers who watched Mr. Rogers' Neighborhood or Barney and Friends tended to get along better with other children than those who didn't. These programs convey the message to children that empathy, compassion, and friendship are important components of a happy life. Children who watch these programs model their behaviors after what they see.

Do unto your child as you want your child to do unto others, says Lerner. If he throws his crayons in anger, calmly insist that he help pick them up– but tell him you understand that he's mad too.

5. Self-sufficiency

By learning to act independently, your child will certainly mature with a strong adequate inner compass to know what she wants as well as to make sound judgments on her own. Possibly one of the most effective quality you can pass on to your child– one that assists him to be patient, accountable, and also self-sufficient– is the capacity to address issues. If your 14-month-old is getting quick-tempered since she cannot have fun with an additional child's plaything, acknowledge her worry, yet encourage her to look for other remedies, suggests Phillips.

Help your child break jobs right into little actions, and afterwards let her master each step on her very own. If she can figure out just how to take down her very own towel, open up the cookie jar, or spread jelly on her gesture, she'll feel more confident and autonomous concerning tackling larger tasks around your home.

You can likewise assist construct self-direction by providing your child age-appropriate things to do. At age 1, that may indicate finding out to eat with a spoon, as well as a year later on, placing on a loose-fitting t-shirt. Make things as easy as possible– get shoes with self-fasteners as opposed to laces, for instance– and be prepared to aid when essential. If your child seriously wants a cookie, take her up so she can open the cupboard, order the bundle, as well as select one out by herself.

One of the most effective methods for your child to discover self-reliance is by modeling your behavior. If you're having problem, say, assembling your new computer system, talk to yourself out loud, strolling yourself with the steps, so your child can see you undergoing the procedure of addressing the trouble.

While you're at it, don't forget to foster your child's individuality. Remember that it's important to solicit and acknowledge her opinions. When shopping, ask your toddler to select a shirt from a choice of two.

Problem is, teaching these qualities can be time-consuming– allowing children resolve their own troubles requires time– and that's something parents just don't have. You'll be helping your child more if you resist jumping in and doing things for her. That added minute will pay off in the coming years.

BEING THE PARENT YOUR CHILD NEEDS

While parents aren't expected to be "ideal," it really isn't generally that made complex to increase happy, well-adjusted children.

Children need love. Children need borders. Children require somebody to respect as well as learn from.

Your key duty, as parents, is to lead by instance– modeling the type of actions that you want your children to take on.

Ending up being a role model, naturally, often means taking a close, honest look at exactly how you live your very own life.

This kind of soul-searching can be uneasy, sometimes, however it's absolutely required for the well-being of your child.

If you're ready to step up to the plate, here are ways to lead by instance, assisting your children to develop personality and self-regard, and also revealing them: "This is what awesomeness looks like."

Be your best. Role-modeling is everything when it comes to your children. Your children pay attention to every little thing you claim and do, and they imitate your activities and also words. Bear in mind exactly how easily they are influenced. Be your finest.

Care for yourself. Being your finest starts with taking excellent care of yourself– obtaining sufficient sleep, making time to work out, consuming excellent food, as well as finding healthy methods to take care of negative emotions without snapping.

Diminishing yourself by frequently placing other individuals' needs very first is not a good move. That's not the sort of future you want for your child– so don't design it, yourself.

Be reliable. You don't intend to elevate a child who lets people down– so ensure to model stability.

That suggests coming through for your child (" I guaranteed that we 'd likely to the park after you cleaned up your space, so allows go!") as opposed to letting job or various other obligations constantly precede. It additionally means coming through for good friends, home, colleagues, and also every person else in your life.

Check in with yourself. "Checking in" to review your very own behavior is a stunning practice– as well as it's healthy and balanced for your child to see and also hear you doing it, also.

You can open up conversations with your child by claiming points like:

Lately, I've been believing, I may be enjoying way too much TELEVISION.

I'm feeling a bit worn out. I assume that I require to start eating far better food.

Today I really felt so mad! I assume it's time for me to take a look at just how I manage conflict with others.

Welcome your child into the conversation to share some points that he or she would certainly such as to enhance or explore. By doing this, you're enhancing the concept that being an outstanding individual is an ongoing process. There's always room to learn and also expand!

We live in an age where getting rid of a "close friend" from your life can occur at the touch of a switch. Show your child what real loyalty looks like– showing up to help a friend in a time of need or sticking with a local business owner who has served your family for years, instead of hopping over to the newest cheap-o mega-store.

Be attentive. Your role is to be a parent. Which means being attentive and making sure that your child isn't in harm's way– even if your child thinks you're "annoying."

You can say something like:

" You are so valuable to me, and it's my obligation to ensure that you're healthy and balanced and also secure, constantly. I wish that one day, you'll recognize why it's my obligation to be so mindful and also to care for the people I like. I really hope that someday, if you have children, you'll be worried and attentive, too."

Children are naturally trusting, and they look eagerly to their surroundings for role models. Show them what it looks like to have a healthy skepticism and to "follow your instincts."

At a car dealership, you could privately turn to your child say:

" These salesmen are saying that this is the very best sell town, however I have a hunch they might not be correct. Let's check out some other car dealerships. It's crucial to trust your gut."

Fess up when you've behaved inappropriately. When you behave inappropriately– say, yelling angrily at your spouse because you're hungry and grumpy– don't make excuses.

It's healthy for your child to see examples of taking responsibility for their actions– as well as carrying out "repercussions" to fix inappropriate behavior.

" I wanted to go out for a jog, today, but I yelled at your father and that triggered a big fight. Instead, we're most likely to stay home and spend some time chatting, together. We're most likely to find out a strategy to make sure that this doesn't happen once again."

Carry out repercussions when your child behaves wrongly. Several parents are hesitant to apply repercussions when a child breaks a policy, yet consistency is required.

When your child does something unacceptable, it's important that you implement an appropriate consequence. Children tend to thrive on consistency and reliability.

Begin now. The habits that children develop at a very early age tend to remain with them as they age. Since bad habits can be hard to damage, among the most effective things you can do for your children, from the first day, is to design behavior that positively forms their character and also values, and furnishes them to live liable, productive lives.

The earlier, the better. The even more regular, the much better.

That said, regardless of what age your children are, it's never ever far too late to start to design the actions you desire your children to. embrace–increasing amazing children who mature to come to be outstanding grownups!

PROVEN WAYS TO TREAT OPPOSITIONAL DEFIANT DISORDER (INTRODUCING ALTERNATIVE BEHAVIORS)

Implementing an actions intervention strategy to lower or stop a difficult actions is one point. Yes, but there is likewise an opportunity that your child will simply learn another difficult actions to obtain him the same outcome. Teaching the alternative behavior, in a method, can make the "unlearning" of the tough actions much faster.

There are four reasons children may take part in challenging actions: either to obtain something she or he desires (access), to get out of doing something they don't want (getaway), to get attention, or due to the fact that the behavior itself really feels good or pleases them (self-stimulatory/automatic). The general theme that you will see throughout this post is that the different behavior that you must instruct your child needs to still lead to your child obtaining what they desire (i.e., among the 4 reasons).

Let's say your child screams and also throws things when they are done with their dinner. Your child is attempting to leave something– the table. What might you educate your child to do instead of shouting as well as tossing? You can possibly show your child to "effectively" communicate when they are done whether it be signing "all done" with their hands, stating "all done," giving an "all done" laminated picture to a grown-up at the table, or some other mode of interaction based on your child's collection of skills. Initially, assist your child when you start to see the indicators of them being all done by directing them through the physical motions of interacting (i.e., exchanging a picture or finalizing), or modeling the words they should use. Gradually discolor this aid until they are doing it on their own, without participating in the difficult habits.

The same approaches should be utilized for the various other "functions" of actions, or when your child involves in challenging habits for various other factors. It is vital to offer your child cookies every time they ask when they are initial knowing as this will certainly be the trick to lowering the challenging habits of climbing up on the counter.

For attention-based difficult behaviors, one way to tackle this is to figure out what you believe your child ought to be doing rather of the improper behavior. Of course, considering your child's collection of skills first is crucial when figuring out what replacement habits to teach.

When your child engages in challenging actions because it feels good, a bit more thought has to be placed into the alternate behavior. If your child involves in repeating words/phrases or just vocalizing noises that are not socially appropriate, enabling your child to engage in these behaviors in a specific setting (e.g., their room) as well as showing them to ask for "chatting in my area" or something similar may assist to obtain control of where they might engage in this behavior.

Many children with autism use improper behaviors in order to get their demands fulfilled. Whatever behaviors the child is showing, will continue to take place because on some level, the habits "works" for the child. In other words, there is some need that this actions is fulfilling.

The three (3) major "demands".

The three major "needs" that the unfavorable behavior might relate to (functions of the habits) are:

1. Gaining attention or preferred items.

2. Avoiding or escaping a circumstance or a demand.

3. The actions they are engaging in really feels excellent.

The very first step when faced with an problematic action is to attempt to figure out why the child is responding the way he is. Of course, we all have "off" days due to a variety of reasons, however, if an problematic actions is consistent, there's a relationship between the habits as well as what occurs prior to and/or after it that is creating the behavior to proceed. The task of a behavior expert is to figure out what that relationship is so that an appropriate strategy can be established to address the behavior.

In order to determine this relationship, it is essential to really spend time tape-recording and observing what occurs right before (antecedent) and also right after (repercussion) the actions. The information recorded,must be exactly what behavior was observed, not an impact of what triggered it. It's additionally practical to create the specific times of day the behavior each actions is happening and also various other setting events to help determine if there is a pattern of the actions.

When the information is collected for a period of time, the team reviews the information to look for patterns in the events happening before and after the behavior. For example,say that when the group looked at Sam's behaviors, the observed that there was not any type of consistency with concerns to what happened after the actions. (antecedent occasion) as well as the tantrum (actions).

On the other hand, probably the information gathered showed a different relationship. Maybe one person asked, "What do you desire?" another asked, "Are you hungry?"and also, a thirdopened up the refrigerator and also provided Sam his juice. The only point that corresponded was that after the temper tantrum occurred (consequence), everybody revealed Sam various items untilthey located the one he wanted as well as he stopped crying. This would indicate the relationship is between the habits and also obtaining the preferred product.

As soon as the connection is identified, a strategy can be developed to deal with the trouble habits. Behavior reduction treatments typically include 1) manipulation of what comes prior to the behavior (antecedent events), 2) removal of the reinforcer that is maintaining the behavior (termination) 3),teaching the child a replacement behavior by supplying a higher density of support for the alternate behavior (differential support of different actions). The objective is to instruct the child a substitute behavior (talking, signing or exchanging pictures/objects) to serve the same function as the adverse behavior. The improper and proper habits in this scenario are called a "reasonable pair."

Rather, the team might choose to right away open up the refrigerator and also give Sam some selections of products he could desire. As he go for an item, the team might instantly motivate Sam to utilize the word, sign, picture or things to ask for the one he desires. For requesting this means, the team may plan to give him even more of the requested product than he typically gets (differential support of alternative actions).

Sam undoubtedly has a hostility to listening to those words most likely due to something he didn't like taking place at the exact same time he heard those words. Or probably the team would certainly decide to simply "pair" those words with reinforcement by claiming them while Sam was engaged in a favored activity yet not needing an action. While enjoying the Sam's favored video clip with him, they may say, "What do you want?"

Reinforcement, by its meaning, is what takes place after the habits happens (variable ratio reinforcement schedule). In fact, if the child was provided what he desired (enhanced) every time he throws a tantrum (continuous reinforcement routine) prior to our efforts to intervene, it would really be simpler for us to snuff out the behavior. Unlike the case of the port equipment, our behavior of placing money in would stop rather swiftly!

When we first start denying accessibility to the reinforcer (termination), it's crucial to understand that we normal see a rise in the child's behavior. In this case, Sam's temper tantrum might intensify or last longer than common. This is called a "termination ruptured" and will certainly lessen quite rapidly as long we correspond in not allowing accessibility to the reinforcer. An example of this extremeoutburst would be if the individual who expected to obtain candy from the candy machine struck the machine or kicked it a few times in effort to obtain the support he was made used to obtaining. It's essential to "ride out" behavior ruptured as opposed to assume it suggests our treatment isn't working.

In some cases, also after a habits is stopped by not permitting access to the reinforcer (extinction), the child will suddenly show the same behavior once more. Once more, it's very crucial that the very same treatment be complied with to not permit the child accessibility to the reinforcer. If not, the actions might come back completely stressed as well as be much more resistant to termination in the future!

Because of the value of consistency when taking care of a child's habits, it's essential that everyone working or interacting with the child be informed of the strategy. It's usually best to discuss the procedures very plainly so everybody comprehends what to do. In addition, it's ideal to clarify why the treatments are being made use of as well as the value of every person responding in a consistent way. If the behavior is reinforced often and not others, it will be a growing number of resistance to end it. As an example, let's say that Sam's parents had striven to instruct Sam to make use of indications to ask for things, yet then a babysitter came over to spend a night. This sitter really did not understand anything about Sam's background of tantrums or the procedures made use of to quit them, so, when Sam went to the refrigerator and also began crying, the babysitter began showing him things untilshe identified what he wanted. All the work the parents had done to snuff out the outburst would certainly be lost, and actually, the habits would be extra immune to endingsince the outburst was again strengthened!

Basically, we must educate the child that making use of pictures/objects, indicators or words is the way to connect his requires as well as desires. As part of this, we must additionally show him that unfavorable habits will certainly not be successful in obtaining his demands fulfilled!

PROVEN WAYS TO TREAT OPPOSITIONAL DEFIANT DISORDER (SET BOUNDARIES)

Part of aiding our children to be the very best they can be, occasionally implies explaining things they can do in different ways. They could not constantly enjoy to receive the information– they're no different from the rest of us who are like that. There's a distinction though– a huge distinction– in between feedback that's given with charitable intent and that which fractures the child's self-concept or self-esteem. Anything that creates pity, embarrassment, or the "shrinking" of a child is hazardous.

We're here to grow our children, to help them discover flight, as well as to help them browse around anything that could lead them to believe those wings of theirs are damaged. Their wings are never ever broken, yet individuals who touch their lives sometimes are.

It's not constantly simple to withdraw a child from a poisonous grownup, specifically if that grownup is a parent or a teacher, yet there are things we can do to strengthen the guard around them and also teach them the abilities that will certainly shield them permanently– because let's be honest, toxic people will go and come throughout the healthiest of lives and also it's not uncommon for them to latch on to individuals who are kind, charitable, or open.

Self-control seems to be no barrier to their poisonous substance. Occasionally, we will not see them coming as well as the very first we'll understand is that day we wake up as well as the world really feels a little blacker.

Strength and nerve can be found in at the point of closing down to the influence of somebody that's hazardous. It's in everybody to do this, as well as it's up to us to offer our children a lamplight to locate theirs, authorization to utilize it, as well as modeling to reveal them just how.

Points first– is it actually hazardous?

Policy out other explanations for just how your child is feeling. Is your child delicate to an adult's tone or volume or rough manner?

Is it a real situation of being targeted by an adult or is your child consistently disturbing the classor speaking during the lesson. Maintain an eye on things. Remember that one of the devices of the trade for poisonous individuals is to condemn various other individuals for their own messed up practices.

Does the individual involved have all the information?

Are there things taking place at home that might be influencing your child's practices? The majority of people will be pleased to get the details as the last thing a non-toxic person would certainly want to do is to unconsciously cause distress.

If the behavior is hazardous ...

If you've developed that it's not an oversensitivity or anything the child is doing, right here's how to secure the child in your life (as well as you) from individuals who may be little them currently, and against the poisonous ones who may come later on.

First, take out support for the grownup.

We're constantly informed as parents to sustain the teacher, the various other parent, the coach, and this is true yet just like whatever else, there's a limitation. When sustaining the adult becomes sustaining his or her poisonous behavior (the contamination of the child's self-confidence, self-confidence or self-concept), it's time to take out assistance. Allow your child understand that you do not agree with the adult– whether it's an educator, instructor or whoever, and that whatever was said or done ought to not have actually occurred.

How to help them establish strong boundaries between themselves as well as the ones who trigger damage.

A border is the line between what is me as well as what is not me; in between what they assume as well as what I assume. With a solid border, there's an approval that simply because they assume it/feel it/state it/do it/doesn't mean I have to.

We all have a thing around us called a limit, which is a line between ourselves as well as other individuals. You cannot see it however it's there. It's type of like an undetectable forcefield and it's there to secure each of us from the people who really feel poor to be about– not the ones who feel good to be around a lot of the times, but sometimes get grouchy or cross. However, the ones that state mean things or do imply points that you simply don't be worthy of.

You are totally in charge of that forcefield around you. You can decide when it goes up and also when it boils down. You can determine what's allowed in as well as what has to stay out. You're the one in charge and also you'll always be in charge.

Now, it's still vital to listen as well as learn from individuals when they advise you concerning things you need to do differently– it's the trick of being incredible. In some cases however, there may be people that do or state mean points so often that you never ever really feel great when you're around them.

We can't control other people, however, we can control whether we allowed the mean things they do, or say come close sufficient to harm us. Being a child is different– as well as if you're outstanding at it.

Every person is responsible for exactly how they deal with other individuals, including grown-ups and you, yet the person you need to deal with the absolute best is yourself. Occasionally that indicates not listening to what other people may state about you.

Often you have to be your very own hero and secure yourself from being injured by people that don't recognize the rules concerning being kind and also considerate. This is necessary because you're incredible– you're smart, kind, amusing endure as well as strong– and also the globe requires every bit of you.

"Did you understand ...?"

Poisonous behavior is typically automatic. People do it without considering it or taking into consideration that there's a better method to be. That's not an excuse– not an all– however, it can be an important way for your child to more take on the reality that the means a person is treating them really has nothing to do with them at all.

Children will typically have a tendency to assume that adults know what they're doing. Let them know that nobody is excellent– and that when it concerns just how to "be" with individuals, some adults do not recognize what they're doing whatsoever.

Here's how to start the chat:

Did you recognize that a lot of the important things we do are automated? A lot of time, people simply do points due to the fact that it's what they've always done. They do not even think of it.

What this indicates is that when individuals are mean as well as do things that feel bad to you, they haven't stopped to assume that there might be a far better means to do it. Sometimes it's because they have not had any kind of adults in their lives to educate them when they were children, so they mature doing things that aren't that great. The behavior part of their mind does points prior to the kind part of their mind can say, "Hang on a second. You'll hurt a person if you do that to them."

It's important to recognize that individuals' brains can transform. Simply since somebody is mean to you now, does not suggest that individual will constantly be that wayto you– yet you do not have to wait for that to put your defensesup.

No! When you utilize it the rightway, it's the best word in the world.

For such a little word, stating "no" can feel really difficult in some cases but the point is, it can be the bravest, most effective word in the universe. If somebody is asking you to do something that really feels negative, incorrect, or awkward, it's constantly fine to say, "No." It can be a hard word to claim since you could stress regarding what individuals will think of you if you say it. Yet, if they're asking you to do something that really feels bad, then what they think of you currently doesn't matter.

Do not let them change you.

Assist your children to see the value of maintaining their own personality as well as the excellent features of them despite the things that may change them.

There's a bully as well as a hero in all of us and it's vital not to become a bully when you're taking care of bullies. This isn't constantly very easy. You could really feel unfortunate or mad or afraid and wish to harm the individual that has actually injured you– yet you're much better than that. Respecting yourself doesn't imply disrespecting other people. Be kind. Be caring. Be strong. But that does not imply you have to like them.

It's completely fine to forgive individuals that are mean. It's a really hard thing to do, but that doesn't imply you have to accept these individuals back if you do not believe they deserve you. Just comprehend that there are numerous reasons that individuals do unfavorable things, as well as none are as a result of the person you are. You're remarkable. We currently understand that. Mean people weren't born mean. Something happened to transform them in this way. Probably something rather horrible. Simply do not let that happen to you.

Your joy does not rely on what somebody else considers of you.

The fact is, no one will certainly ever recognize whatever is concerning you. If it's someone who claims unfavorable things and also who feels harmful to be around, that sort of person will actually never recognize the best of you and also actually, they aren't worthy to. They'll never ever know just how amusing you are, how kind you are, the remarkable way you think of things, just how brave, strong as well as clever you are, and just how crazy great you are to be around when you trust individuals you're with.

Remain calm

Your child requires to know that you've got this. It's so important not to do anything that might trigger them to really feel as though they need to look after you.

Be their voice

Occasionally we have to be the voice for our children, particularly in relationships where their own is the quieter, softer as well as less effective. When it's time to speak to the adult included, start by being open as well as curious: Is there something my child is doing that he or she needs to enhance? Then, preserve feeling from it and also remain with particular information, "I 'd like to talk with you about something you may not recognize..."

You'll have more possibility of being effective if you can limit the possibility of a defensive reaction. That suggests not going on the strike. You'll intend to, but don't. Stick to the truths. Share the information you have concerning just how the behavior is influencing your child or their capability to work, learn, be: 'When you do [...], [...] happens. I understand that you could not indicate anything by it as well as you might not even realizing it is occurring, but it's simply not obtaining the very best result.

Ask how the individual plans to attend to things for the future. If they aren't prepared to do anything, most likely to greater, if you can, take your child out of their hands– they are not entitled to the influence. No grownup needs to like your child, but if they don't, they need to keep that to themselves and not let the child know. That's a big "Don't argue" to the grownup. No child needs to have to take care of the feelings of an adult.

When it's peer friendships.

Discovering that it's okay to letgo of relationships is such an important part of complete living. Too often we hold on to people who don't deserve us or that prepare to move in a various direction. Not everyone who enters into our lives is suggested to remain and if we can have our children start to think about this when they're young, they'll be a lot a lot more encouraged as well as calculated in their connections when they're older.

Sometimes individuals just aren't able to be the way you would certainly like them to be. There are individuals out there who will certainly enjoy you so much and also like being with you simply the way you are. Also, well as letting go of the people who really feel negative to be around will certainly make space for the ones who feel excellent to be with.

In some cases, individuals with less friends are the most incredible people you can ever meet– it's just that they're waiting for the appropriate individuals to discover them. Being yourself doesn't indicate that there's something wrong with you– it absolutely does not imply that! It suggests that you recognize what's right for you and also you know you deserve someone that makes the effort to discover out the fantastic things concerning you– as well as that is completely amazing.

The most essential things is not to stay with people who are mean since you're frightened of being on your very own. Being by yourself can feel lonesome, yet being around the wrong kind of individuals feels also lonelier, and completely horrible.

PROVEN WAYS TO TREAT OPPOSITIONAL DEFIANT DISORDER (USE POSITIVE REINFORCEMENT)

Positive support is a crucial habit for parents to create since it is so easy to neglect children when they're behaving properly. It is the annoying and turbulent habits we often tend to respond and observe to.

Train yourself to reveal to your children that you appreciate their efforts and that you acknowledge things they achieve.

Making use of positive reinforcement is a very easy way to nix habits issues. The use of positive reinforcers can assist you motivate your child to do daily jobs you require her to perform. Getting dressed, cleaning her teeth, as well as also getting to bed on schedule are just a few of the things that can be boosted using positive reinforcement.

Any kind of reward or motivation you give your child that leads to enhancing the behavior you want your child to do is a positive reinforcer.

" Education is instructing our children to desire the right things."– Plato

Positive reinforcement is just one of four (4) types of reinforcement in operant conditioning theory of human behavior and among many approaches to parenting. It is planned to urge a desired behavior by presenting incentives quickly after the occurrence as well as consequently raising the probability of repeating.

It's like the basic concept of positive psychology which emphasizes the demand to concentrate on what is great in human nature. Also much like positive psychology does not assert to represent a full sight of human psychology, using positive reinforcement alone does not produce an efficient design for parenting, yet is rather complementary to it, while taking a main stage in many contemporary versions of positive parenting reviewed below.

"The objective of Positive Psychology is to militarize a modification in psychology from an obsession only with fixing the worst points in life to likewise constructing the best top qualities in life."– Martin Seligman

Positive reinforcement can be made use of to encourage habits we intend to enhance, like your child brushing her teeth without a difficulty, or to compensate your child for practicing brand-new skills and also can motivate him to proceed, like putting onshoes or loading a dishwashing machine.

Lasting Positive Reinforcement

For positive reinforcement to be efficient and also of durable worth, it may require a modification of behavior for the parent as long as it is planned to change the habits of a child. Some of us will have to develop a strength not only to criticize versus commend but also to congratulate well.It might not feel natural at first.

For numerous parents the all-natural propensity to deal with and repair behavior issues was implanted in their own childhood as well as is usually well-intentioned, but over-reliance on this technique robs us of the many possibilities to see what our children currently achieve.

"There is no such thing as a perfect parent. Simply be a genuine one."– Sue Atkins

As research in positive feelings by Barbara Fredrickson shows that the ratio of 5 to 1 in positive to unfavorable feelings adds to happiness, a comparable ratio of positive reinforcementto other forms of corrective measures (suchnegative reinforcement) should also generate far better results, as well as inevitably better parents and also children

Following this design, the use of positive reinforcement, as an example, should outweigh circumstances of criticism 5 to 1 to boost positive effects and also well-being, both in children and their parents.

Growth, Development, as well as Self-Worth

One of the most important element of efficient praise is to match the behavior not the person. Professor Carol Dweck of Stanford University discusses how commending the effort versus the individuality of the child sustains a development way of thinking and also a feeling of self-worth.

Her widely known book *Mindset: The New Psychology of Success*, which discusses the roots of innate inspiration, worries the importance of focusing on the child's capacity to pursue objectives as well as dedication to learning brand-new skills which is within his control over integral high qualities like individuality which are an offered as well as often hard to change.

" Your children need you above all to like them for that they are, not to spend your entire time attempting to remedy them."– Bill Ayers

Affection is likewise extremely vital in how we express our approval, according to Dr. John Gottman, a long-time scientist who researches favorable home dynamics. His publications *The Heart of Parenting: How to Raise an Emotionally Intelligent Child* and also *Meta-Emotions: How Families Communicate Emotionally,* provides a checklist of many functional tools for improving emotional connection with our children even in the hardest of moments and remind us that expressions of warmth and concern creates trust and also enhances closeness.

Examples of Positive Reinforcement at Use

General examples of positive reinforcement can be located almost everywhere, from pet dog training methods to worker benefits and also award programs (Daniels, 2016). Positivereinforcers are likewise extensively utilized in schoolsystems and also childcare facilities to attract children to perform a task, find out a brand-new ability, or show a desired behavior much more regularly or in a timely manner. It can be also properly be replicated in the house.

A few of the apparent instances of positive reinforcement used in schools that can quickly equate to parenting circumstances include:

- Compliments and also recognition

- Public praise, favorable notes to instructors and parents

- Pats on the back, smiles, hand-shakes, and also high-fives

- Being the educator's helper or selection of classroom tasks

- Reading, making crafts, playing sporting activities, or other recommended task with a special person

- Extra credit or bonus offer features on schoolwork

- Posting work in a location of honor

- A homework-free evening

- Choice of activities

- Time or lunch with somebody special

- Increased recess time

Children of all ages react well to praise as they wish to please their parents and more often wish to be viewed as making great choices. When we commend positive actions and choices, we encourage our children to duplicate them. Catch your child in the act of being "great" as well as when your she is behaving in a way you like, offer her some positive comments.

As an example, you can tell her, "I truly like the way you're keeping all the blocks on the table," which functions better than awaiting the blocks to come crashing down prior to you taking notice and also say, "Be careful!" Since it informs children particularly what they're doing well, this form of positive comments are understood as detailed praise. Our lives are full of uncertainties as children's writer Shel Silverstein that explains in his brief poem:

When the light is green you go,
When the light is red you quit
When the light is blue,
 But what do you
With orange as well as lavender spots

Bear in mind to make a minimum of five (5) positive comments for every negative reaction due to the fact that if children have a selection in between no attention or negative attention, they'll typically go for obtaining a raising of out you.

Detailed supports are powerful incentives. Also, young adults, that could appear self-dependent, still desire and require your approval. When you see your older child's responsible choices you urge her to maintain acting that way. But be sensitive to the fact that young adults commonly like you to be commended independently instead of in front of their close friends (Belsky, 2008).

With young adults, offering a lot more privileges or increasing responsibilities can likewise be a very efficient kind of reward. We have to want to talk about and adjust guidelines as our children reveal better sense of responsibility as they grow older, for example, by extending a child's curfew.

Using Positive Reinforcement to Change Children's Behavior

One of the most crucial things to remember when utilizing positive reinforcement to change behavior is to bear in mind the last time we attempted to alter one of our very own routines. It simply takes time, determination and patience.

Frequency as well as Consistency

When utilizing positive support to alter behavior uniformity, immediacy as well as regularity are extremely essential. When a child is learning a brand-new ability supplying reinforcement right away as well as usually keeps them motivated and committed. Below is where reinforcement schedules come in handy.

Continuous schedule of reinforcers presented regularly after every event of wanted actions while not easy to preserve represents operant conditioning at its most intense and also efficient.

Supports can likewise be offered at a taken care of ratio after a particular variety of events or repaired interval after agreed upon amount of time.

Finally, variable schedules can be presented when where we offer incentives less regularly as the moment takes place so as to avoid the reliance on benefits in favor of promoting of internal motivation to carry out the desired behavior.

Monitoring progression is also important so adjustments can be made based upon child's preference for the type of rewards. Soliciting child's preferences can itself enhance inspiration by presenting a choice as well as a result cultivating a feeling of autonomy.

Checking for satiation can aid to prevent reinforcers from lessening in power. Below we can use more selection by switching over the reward systems, by readjusting the sessions of supports from constant to periodic, specifically after the wanted behavior is established.

What Rewards Are Best?

The sort of incentives we provide is additionally extremely crucial and also relies on the context as some of them like all-natural reinforcers happen naturally therefore of child's habits as well as may not need our intervention.

All-natural reinforcers in form of good qualities or a feeling of self-satisfaction for a job well done are most effective as they support self-confidence, sense of firm as well as rise inherent motivation.

Social reinforcers like acknowledgment or authorization of others that can be expressed via matches, support, and particular praise are also really powerful as they communicate approval as well as belonging.

Token reinforcers which are used instead of substantial rewards can likewise be effective in urging development towards objectives as they can be used quickly and are an efficient visual representation of continuous effort. A child can make factors or accumulate token which they can then sell for something of value to them.

Concrete benefits can be utilized to kickstart inspiration, but fulfillment in the job well done should be stressed. We wish to make use of rewards to bring back motivation not to make them the item of search, so the children don't become dependent on rewards.

If we're attempting to extinguish benefits, we want to wait before we compensate by gradually reducing the regularity or by expanding the length of intervals in between the introductions of positive reinforcers to separate the task from the incentive (Lynch, 2017).

Positive Reinforcement Checklists

Below is a soup to nuts positive reinforcement list (PDF) with recommendations for reinforcement schedules that can be utilized for younger children. It's geared toward teachers yet can be applied just as efficiently in your home.

Positive Reinforcement Children

While sensory, social or natural reinforcers are of more enduring worth, when it involves younger children concrete reinforcements might be made use of to include selection, boost the immediacy as well as regularity. Concrete rewards need to always be connected to actions as well as values we are trying to promote.

Several of the valuable techniques for use with more youthful children is connecting via photos and presenting reinforcers briefly to encourage search as hidden can usually run out mind.

Does it Work?

The short answer is yes it does, but there are caveats to making use of favorable reinforcement properly since they stand for only a part of what comprises favorable discipline.

According to Jane Nelsen Ed.D., that had been writing on positive parenting since 1980s, favorable self-control tools remove the demand for punishment as well as protect against the potential damages that can be triggered by permissive parenting.

Her positive self-control design is based upon kindness and suppleness at the same time. It encourages parents to provide opportunities for children to establish in locations that will certainly reinforce their assumptions and skills in core aspects of life by asking interested questions and entailing children is establishing limitations. The seven core understandings and also skills we must be fostering in children, according to Nelsen, include:

- Sense of company as well as individual capability that child can deal with most points in life.

- Strong understanding of one's relevance in key partnership and feeling genuinely needed and also contributing.

- Belief in being able to influence what occurs to them as well as sense of individual power far from discovered vulnerability.

- Intrapersonal abilities that involve self-understanding, psychological knowledge, and also self-discipline.

- Interpersonal skills of interaction, energetic listening, compassion, participation, discussing as well as sharing,

- Systemic skills of obligation, flexibility, adaptability and stability.

- Judgement abilities as well as the capability to review scenarios in accordance with their values.

What are the Benefits and Advantages?

The benefits of positive reinforcement remain in step with what positive psychology educates us regarding cultivating positive state of mind and also concentrating on what is great in individuals. While our natural tendency is to correct, take care of, and addressing problems, it usually does not create a much more efficient approach and often tends to alienate those we're attempting to help.

Many would certainly agree that it is much more pleasurable to be commended as well as value our children when they already do well, instead of constantly criticizing them. While honesty as well as useful feedback are essential, so is the appropriate balance between appreciation and other type of discipline.

Positive reinforcement additionally permits parents to prevent the long-lasting adverse consequences of punishment which are not constantly immediately visible. With time,punishment develops resentment as well as untrustworthiness, rebellion, and even vengeance which motivates the children to be daring as well as do the opposite of what we ask. Some might pull away into themselves and begin to hide as well as lie, and also in other instances internalize the act of punishment and think of themselves as an evildoer.

" Making the choice to have a child– it's memorable. It is to choose for life to have your heart go walking outside your body."– Elizabeth Stone

As Dr. John Gottman describes, many of the difficult moments when we discipline our children, we are additionally teaching moments that when approached with moderate generosity, it can be used to promote greater connection and also help our children learn from their blunders.

Emotional intelligence goes to the heart of efficient parenting. While handling emotions can be difficult for many adults, it is our job as parents to show as well as model for our children just how to manage and handle frustrating feelings. His approach for emotions mentoring for children suggests that we:

- Describe behavior in regards to what we see as well as only after that claim just how we feel concerning it

- Model actions we desire them to mimic and also do not oppose it e.g. by yelling

- Apologize

- Respect their demands

- Validate their experience

- Help them address problems

- Think before we say no

Many of us originate from family members of inadequate communicators where we were believed that unfavorable feelings were not okay. Gottman reminds us that while not all habits are appropriate, all feelings are normal, also we intend to acknowledge and confirm them to make sure that our children do not learn to define themselves through their wrong actions.

What Happens To a Child Hospitalized for ODD? What Can I Expect?

Having your child hospitalized for a psychological trouble can be a stressful experience. Hospitalization usually is on an emergency basis, often following some sort of extreme event. Parents are frequently exhausted, distressed, and frightened.

If your child remains overnight, you need to go homeand also get some rest. Use this time to pull yourself together, to support your partner and any other children in the home, and simply to take pleasure in some peace for a while.

During a hospital stay, the child may experience the following treatments:

- Group Therapy run by clinical team.
- Individual Therapy with a mental health care professional.
- Home Meetings to prepare the person and the home for the child's return house.
- Time Out if required. If the child ends up being unable to regulate himself, he may be divided from the other individuals. If he seems fierce, he might be put in a "safety area."

Restrictions might be utilized for people that pose a risk to themselves or others. This normally entails leather bands or straps utilized to hold the child in a bed.

CONCLUSION

Although it might not be possible to prevent ODD, acting and also identifying on signs when they initially appear can minimize distress to the child as well as family, and avoid a number of the issues related to the illness. Family members likewise can discover actions to take if signs of relapse (return of signs and symptoms) show up. In addition, providing a nurturing, helpful, and also consistent home environment with a balance of love and suitable strategies may help in reducing signs and symptoms and protect against episodes of defiant behavior.

A child diagnosed with ODD is not immediately going to establish conduct condition. It is essential, nonetheless, for parents to carefully monitor the habits of their child and to seek treatment from a credentialed specialist as early in the child's life as possible.

A child with ODD can be very difficult for parents. These parents need assistance and also understanding. Parents can aid their child with ODD in the following methods:

- Constantly build on the positives, offer the child appreciation and also positive reinforcement when s/he reveals versatility or cooperation.

- Take a break or restif you will make the conflict with your child even worse, not better. This is excellent modeling for your child. If s/he decides to take a break to avoid overreacting, support your child.

- Choose your battles. Given that the child with ODD has problem preventing power struggles, prioritize the important things you desire your child to do. Don't include time for suggesting if you offer your child a time-out in his area for wrongdoing. State "your time will start when you go to your area."

- Establish practical, age ideal limits with consequences that can be enforced continually.

- Maintain rate of interests aside from your child with ODD, to make sure that handling your child does not take all your time and energy. Try to work with as well as get assistance from the other adults (instructors, counsellors, and also partner) managing your child.

- Manage your own stress and anxiety with healthy life choices, such as exercise and also relaxation. Usage reprieve treatment and also other breaks as needed.

Many children with ODD will certainly react to the favorable parenting strategies. Parents may ask their pediatrician or family doctor to refer them to a child/teenage psychiatrist or other qualified mental health and wellness expert that can assist in identifying as well as dealing with ODD and any kind of associated psychological condition.

Do Not Go Yet; One Last Thing To Do

If you enjoyed this book or found it useful, I'd be very grateful if you'd post a short review on Amazon. Your support does make a difference. I read all the reviews personally so I can get your feedback and make this book even better.

Thanks again for your support!

ADHD

A Proven Guide to Managing, Healing, And Coping With ADHD In Children

TABLE OF CONTENTS

WHAT IS ADHD

Attention-deficit Hyperactivity Disorder(ADHD) is one of the most common mental disorders affecting children. ADHD additionally impacts lots of adults. Signs of ADHD consist of inattentiveness (not having the ability to keep focused), hyperactivity (unusually or abnormally active), and impulsivity (rash acts that occur in the minute without thought).

An approximated 8.4 percent of children and also 2.5 percent of adults have ADHD. ADHD is usually initially diagnosed in school-aged children when it brings about disruption in the class or troubles with schoolwork. It can, likewise, impact adults. It is more common among boys than girls.

WHAT DOES IT MEAN TO HAVE ADHD?

Has anybody ever asked you if you have ADHD? Possibly, you've also wondered yourself. The only way to understand it for sure, is to see a physician. That's because the disorder has a variety of possible symptoms and they can easily be confused with those of other conditions, like clinical depression or stress and anxiety.

Not sure whether a doctor should assess you? If a number of these apply, you may need to see a doctor.

1. People say you're absent-minded.

Everyone loses cars and truck keys or jackets from time to time. This happens when you have ADHD. You may hang around looking for glasses, wallets, phones, as well as various other products each day. You may also forget to return calls, space out on paying bills or miss medical consultations.

2. People complain that you do not pay attention.

Most of us lose concentration on a discussion from time to time, specifically, if there's a TV nearby or something else demanding our interest. It takes place typically and also more frequently with ADHD, even when there are no diversions around. Still, ADHD is even more than that.

3. You're typically behind schedule.

Time management is an ongoing challenge when you have ADHD It usually results in missed due dates or appointments unless you deal with preventing that.

4. You have difficulty concentrating.

Issues with interest, mainly focusing for extended periods or taking notice of details, is just one of the characteristics of the problem. Depression, anxiousness, and also addiction problems can likewise take a toll on your ability to focus, as well as many individuals with ADHD have one or more of these problems, too. Your doctor can ask you questions to get to the root of what's causing your attention issues.

5. You leave things undone.

Problems with interest and also memory can be challenging to start or complete developments. Specifically, ones that you know will take a lot of attention to finish. This symptom can indicate depression as well.

6. You had behavior concerns as a child.

You need to have had attention as well as focus troubles as a child to be identified with ADHD as an adult – even if those early signs didn't feature an official diagnosis.

Individuals might have accused you of laziness back in youth. Or they may have thought you had an additional problem like depression or stress and anxiety.

If you were diagnosed with the disorder as a child, you might still have it. The signs change as you age, and also not everybody outgrows it.

7. You lack impulse control.

It is more than tossing a sweet bar right into your cart at the checkout line. It is doing something even though you understand it could have severe repercussions, like running a red light because you believe you can get away with it or otherwise being able to keep the peace when you have something to state, even though you recognize you should.

8. You cannot get organized.

You might discover this more at work. You could have difficulty setting goals, following up on tasks, and meeting project deadlines.

9. You're nervous.

Children with ADHD are typically hyper, but adults are more likely to be fidgety or troubled. You might also talk too much, as well as to interrupt others.

10. You can't control your emotions.

You may be irritable or short-tempered, express frustration usually, feel indifferent or be susceptible to angry outbursts. ADHD can make it tough to handle awkward feelings or follow ideal habits when you're disturbed.

THE VARIOUS TYPES OF ADHD

Comprehending ADHD

Attention deficit disorder (ADHD) is a chronic condition. It primarily influences children, yet can additionally impact adults. It can affect emotions, behaviors, and also the ability to learn.

ADHD is divided into three different types:

1. Inattentive type
2. Hyperactive-impulsive type
3. Combination of both types

Signs and symptoms will determine which sort of ADHD you have. To be identified with ADHD, signs and symptoms have to influence your daily life.

Signs and symptoms can alter over time, so the type of ADHD you have might change as well. ADHD can be a long-lasting obstacle. Medicine and various other therapies can help improve your quality of life.

Three Types Of Symptoms

Each sort of ADHD is tied to several qualities. ADHD is identified by inattentiveness and hyperactive-impulsive actions.

These Behaviors Are Frequently Present In All Types:

Inattentiveness: being sidetracked, having the inadequate concentration and also organizational abilities

Impulsivity: disturbing, risk taking

Hyperactivity: never appearing to slow down, talking as well as fidgeting, problems remaining on task

Everyone is different, so it's usual for two individuals to experience the very same signs in different ways. For example, these behaviors are typically mixed in young boys and also girls. Children may be seen as more hyperactive, as well as girls may be silently unobserving.

Inattentive ADHD

If you have this type of ADHD, you may experience a lot more signs and symptoms of inattention than those of impulsivity as well as hyperactivity. You might battle with impulse control or hyperactivity at times. These aren't the primary attributes of inattentive ADHD.

People who experience inattentiveness commonly:

- Miss details and also are sidetracked quickly
- Get tired rapidly
- Have difficulty concentrating on a solitary task
- Have trouble organizing thoughts and also learning brand-new info
- Lose pencils, papers, or various other things needed to finish a task
- Don't appear to pay attention
- Move slowly and also look as if they're daydreaming
- Refine details much more slowly as well as much less appropriately than others
- Have a problem following directions

More women are detected with inattentive type ADHD than children.

Hyperactive-Impulsive ADHD

This type of ADHD is defined by signs of impulsivity and attention deficit disorder. People with this type can present indications of inattentiveness. However, it's not as significant as the various other symptoms.

People that are impulsive or hyperactive frequently:

- Squirm, fidget, or feel restless
- Have difficulty sitting still
- Talk continuously
- Touch as well as play with objects, even when inappropriate to the task at hand
- Have trouble engaging in quiet tasks
- Are regularly "on the move"
- Are impatient
- Act out of turn and also don't think of repercussions of actions
- Spout out answers and also inappropriate remarks

Children with hyperactive-impulsive type ADHD can be an interruption in the classroom. They can make discovery more challenging on their own and even other students.

Combination ADHD

If you have the mix type, it indicates that your signs and symptoms do not exclusively fall within the inattentive or hyperactive-impulsive behavior. Instead, a mix of signs and symptoms from both of the categories is displayed.

Many people, with or without ADHD, experience some level of unobserving or spontaneous behavior. Yet it's extra dangerous in individuals with ADHD. The behaviors occur frequently as well as interferes with just how you function at home, school, work, and also in social circumstances.

The Central Institute of Mental Health clarifies that many children have combination type ADHD. The most usual symptom in preschool-age children is hyperactivity.

CAUSES OF ADHD

The reason for ADHD in your child can be traced back to family members. The condition is genetically based, which in simple terms, implies your child may have been predisposed due to your genetics. Even though conditions in your home or school can add to it, they are not considered ADHD reasons.

There have been lots of scientific analyses that link physical attributes to the source of ADHD. These include genetic makeup, absorbing toxic active ingredients, trauma to the brain, and responses to some artificial additive.

The make-up of your genetics:

Check out other members of your household. Did you recognize that even though three to five percent of children are identified with ADHD, 25 percent of an ADHD child's relatives will certainly additionally have the condition? Scientific researchers have also disclosed specific genes that have been linked to the root cause of ADHD!

Toxic components:

If you consumed alcohol or made use of tobacco products while you were expecting, and also you have an ADHD child, researches have indicated a possible link. A fetus will certainly absorb these poisonous compounds, which certainly cannot be excellent. If your child has been around old buildings, he may have been revealed to lead poisoning. Several of these toxic ingredients have been labeled as possible ADHD causes. When I was growing up on an farm, my Dad subjected me to DDT, which is currently outlawed in the USA. Possibly, that added to my ADHD, and then my boy's.

Brain injury:

Most children, fortunately, don't come under this category; however, specific sorts of mental trauma can bring on ADHD signs. Scientific studies had shown that when an ADHD child and a non-ADHD child had brain scans or an MRI, there were some distinctions in some regions of the mind. This would seem to show that the brain has something to do with the source of ADHD.

Food additives:

About 10 percent of ADHD children show minimized signs when their sugar and additive intake has been reduced. Currently, right here is somewhat of a shock. While a lot of us, including me, tend to associate sugar with attention deficit disorder, there was no difference when children were given either sugar or a sugar replacement. That suggests that sugar doesn't contribute to ADHD signs.

Given that a lot of individuals have it in their heads that sugar triggers ADHD symptoms, they may see more signs after a child has some sugar. Studies reveal that moms and dads that believe that their children have been provided sugar (when they have been offered a substitute) are just as most likely to state that ADHD signs have worsened as parents of children that are given actual sugar.

Even if it is only considered, a reduction in sugar consumption (or high fructose) can be beneficial.

A recent study has discovered that preservatives and also food coloring, which can be found in soft drinks as well as fast food, significantly increase hyperactivity in children. So, make sure you see what they are taking into their bodies.

Remember, ADHD triggers children to act in unacceptable means. However, it doesn't need to be this approach. It is an extremely treatable problem. There are prescription drugs that work for the signs, natural remedies that attack the origin of the condition, nutritional control, and behavioral therapy. Do your study, and after that, do what is in your child's best interest.

ADHD SIGNS AND SYMPTOM

To assist you to recognize when your child may have attention deficit hyperactivity disorder, here are some ADHD indicators you should understand:

1) Do you observe your child having difficulty in schooltasks and other activities? The inability to concentrate as well as take note of instructions can result in reduced grades. Children with ADHD also tend to stay clear of working on challenging tasks and try to make excuses whenever they need to do them.

2) Does it appear as if you're always searching for things that your child has lost? Among the ADHD signs are forgetfulness and disorganization. Children with ADHD typically lose things, fail to remember to do homework, and leave their books at school.

3) Do you find your child always daydreaming? Those with ADHD commonly seem not to listen when they are talked to.

4) Is it tough for your child to sit still? Fidgeting and also uneasiness prevail ADHD indications amongst children as they have a tough time remaining in their seats.

5) Does your child disrupt other children in his class due to too much talking? Children with ADHD have a hard time keeping silent, even in situations where they are expected to do so.

6) Does your child act as if an electric motor runs him? Continuously running, jumping, as well as climbing, are also ADHD indicators. Children with ADHD have all this pent-up power that requires to be released through activities like sports.

7) Is your child fond of blurting out a solution to questions that are not yet asked? Spontaneity is one of the ADHD warning signs, and also, this can be possibly dangerous. For instance, they might do something like cross the street without looking.

8) Does your child discover it hard waiting in line for his turn? Children with ADHD often have this trouble, and they likewise interrupt other people who are speaking or in the middle of doing something.

These are ADHD indications that could prompt you to seek specialist help and assessment. Know that there are various therapy options available to you that are more secure and also even more affordable than prescription drugs.

The Four Warning Signs of ADHD Symptoms In Toddlers

Children with ADHD do show signs and symptoms EARLY in their lives. Some parents are worried when their children seem to be a lot more spontaneous and also hyperactive compared with others at the very same age.

Here are a few of the signs and symptoms that children with ADHD may display:

1. Sleeplessness. Some children 2 or 3 years of age are not good sleepers. Children with attention deficiency hyperactivity disorder are a lot more likely to have rest troubles than others, for example, waking up a lot more often throughout the night, and also having difficulty falling asleep.

2. Severe hyper activeness: restless, running around non-stop until too tired to move, and ruining things. I bet these have taken place for most of our young children. However, children with ADHD present these behaviors a lot more frequently and also exceptionally.

3. Inattentiveness: Inattentiveness is just one of the most ordinary signs and symptoms of ADHD. Children with this problem are reported to be much more easily tired at games and toys and are frequently distracted.

4. Hypersensitivity: how do you recognize if your child is hypersensitive? Well, look for the following signs. Do they refuse to put on the clothing of a specific material? Do they have aversions to foods of a particular texture? Some parents complain that their children just won't put on denim trousers because of the hard textiles. My very own child declined to eat bananas and eggs, considering that he was much less than one year of age.

If your young children have revealed the above indications for a minimum of six months, it is encouraged that you speak to their doctor regarding their condition.

When it comes to treatments for this neuro-behavioral problem, prescribed drugs might not be appropriate for extremely young children because of the possible harsh adverse effects.

GETTING AN ACCURATE DIAGNOSIS OF ADHD

Identifying ADHD: What you need to recognize

Are you quickly sidetracked, hopelessly chaotic, or regularly absent-minded and questioning if attention deficit disorder (ADHD) is responsible? Do you take a look at your rambunctious, restless child, and also believe it might be ADHD? Before you leap to conclusions, remember that identifying ADHD isn't somewhat that simple. By themselves, none of the signs and symptoms of attention deficiency disorder are irregular. Most individuals feel scattered, unfocused, or agitated, sometimes. Also, chronic hyperactivity or distractibility is not always equivalent to ADHD.

There is no solitary clinical, physical, or another test for identifying ADHD, previously called ADD. To determine if you or your child has ADHD, a doctor or other health and wellness professionals will certainly need to be entailed, as well as you can expect them to make use of a variety of different tools: a list of signs and symptoms, response to questions concerning past and existing troubles, or a medical examination to eliminate other causes for signs and symptoms.

Keep in mind that the signs of ADHD, such as inattentiveness as well as hyperactivity, can be confused with various other disorders as well as medical problems, consisting of discovering handicaps as well as emotional issues, which require different treatments. Just because it looks like ADHD does not indicate it is, so getting a comprehensive analysis and medical diagnosis is essential.

Making the ADHD medical diagnosis

ADHD looks different in everyone, so there is a wide variety of criteria to help health and wellness experts reach a medical diagnosis. It is essential to be open as well as sincere with the expert performing your analysis to ensure that he or she can get to one of the most precise conclusions.

To obtain an ADHD medical diagnosis, you or your child should display a combination of intense ADHD characteristic symptoms, namely hyperactivity, impulsivity, or inattentiveness. The mental health specialist analyzing the trouble will certainly additionally check out the following variables:

How extreme are the symptoms? To be identified with ADHD, the symptoms have to harm you or your child's life. Generally, people who have

ADHD have significant issues in one or more locations of their life, such as their career, funds, or household responsibilities.

When did the symptoms begin? Given that ADHD starts in childhood years, the physician or specialist will consider precisely how very early the symptoms appeared. If you are an adult, can you trace the signs back to your childhood?

The length of time the symptoms been troubling you or your child? Signs need to have been going on for a minimum of six months before ADHD can be detected.

When and also where do the signs and symptoms appear? The signs of ADHD must exist in numerous setups, such as in the house and even school. If the signs only show up in one atmosphere, it is not likely that ADHD is at fault.

Usual signs and symptoms of ADHD

<u>Signs of inattentiveness</u>

- Often fails to give close attention to information or makes mistakes
- Commonly has problem maintaining focus while completing jobs or partaking in tasks

- Often does not seem to listen when spoken to directly
- Usually does not follow through with instructions as well as fails to finish schoolwork or work environment obligations
- Commonly has trouble organizing tasks and also activities
- Usually avoids, disapprove of or is reluctant to take part in jobs that require continual psychological effort
- Loses products necessary for jobs or activities
- Is easily distracted by nonessential stimulations
- Is usually absent-minded in daily tasks

Signs and symptoms of hyperactivity and also impulsivity

- Typically fidgets with or taps hands and feet, or squirms in seat
- Commonly leaves the position in scenarios when staying seated is anticipated
- Frequently unable to play or engage in leisure activities quietly
- Often runs and also climbs up in situations where it is improper (in adolescents or adults, might be limited to feeling uneasy).

- Is often "on the go," acting as if "driven by an electric motor."
- Commonly blurts out responses before concern has been completed.
- Typically has difficulty waiting their turn.
- Frequently interrupts or invades others.
- Typically talks excessively.

Discovering an expert who can identify ADHD

Certified professionals trained in detecting ADHD can consist of medical psychologists, medical professionals, or scientific, social workers. Choosing an expert can appear confusing. The following actions can aid you to locate the appropriate person to assess you or your child:

1. Get suggestions.

Specialists and good friends you depend on may refer you to a specific specialist. Ask questions concerning their choice as well as check out their suggestions.

2. Do your research.

Figure out the specialist qualification as well as the academic degrees of the professionals you are exploring. Preferably, talk with former people as well as customers, and also learn what their experience was like.

3. Feel secure.

Feeling comfortable with the expert is an integral part of selecting the best person to review you. Attempt to be yourself, ask concerns, and also be honest with the specialist. You might require to speak with a couple of professionals before finding the person that is finest for you.

4. Check rates as well as an insurance policy.

Discover how much the professional will undoubtedly charge as well as if your medical insurance will cover part or every one of the ADHD analysis. Some insurance plan cover assessment for ADHD from one type of specialist, yet not from another.

Detecting ADHD in adults.

Many people only discover that they have ADHD actually when they become adults. Some learn after their children obtain a medical diagnosis. As they end up being enlightened regarding the problem, they likewise understand that they have it. For others, the signs lastly surpass their coping skills, triggering substantial adequate issues in their daily life that they look for aid. If you recognize the symptoms and signs of ADHD in yourself, set up a visit with a psychological wellness professional for an analysis. Once you make that first visit, feeling somewhat anxious regarding it is normal.

If you recognize what to anticipate, the process for reviewing ADHD isn't complicated or scary. Several professionals will begin by asking you to fill in and return questionnaires before an assessment. You'll probably be asked to call a person near to you that will certainly additionally participate in several of the evaluation. To establish if you have ADHD, you can anticipate the specialist conducting the assessment to do any type of or all of the following:

- Ask you about your symptoms, consisting of how long they've been troubling you as well as any troubles they've triggered in the past.
- Administer ADHD examinations, such as symptom lists and also attention-span examinations.
- Speak with a relative or somebody close to you about your symptoms.
- Offer you a medical exam to eliminate other physical causes for the signs.

Should I be tested for adult ADHD?

- If you have substantial problems with any of the following categories, you might want to get assessed for ADHD:
- Work or occupation: shedding or stopping work frequently.
- Job or school: not performing up to your ability or capacity.
- Daily jobs: inability to do family duties, pay bills promptly, organize things.
- Relationships: failing to remember important things, having difficulty completing jobs, getting upset over small issues.
- Emotions: experiencing recurring stress as well as fear because you don't satisfy objectives or meet responsibilities.

Detecting ADHD in children.

When looking for a diagnosis for your child, having a "team attitude" might aid. You are not alone, as well as with the help of others. You can get to the bottom of your child's battles. Together with specialists trained in diagnosing ADHD, you can aid produce a swift and also accurate analysis that results in treatment.

Your role as a parent.

When looking for a diagnosis for your child, you are your child's ideal supporter, as well as the most crucial source of support. As moms and dads in this procedure, your roles are both emotional as well as practical. Here are some things that you can do:

- You can need psychological assistance for your child throughout the analysis procedure.
- Guarantee that your child sees the best professional and also get a second opinion if required.
- Provide unique and handy information for doctors/specialists, including open and also honest answers to questions about your child's history and existing adjustment.
- Demonstrate the speed and accuracy of the analysis.

The Physician's Or Expert's Function.

Usually, more than one specialist examines a child for ADHD signs. Physicians, medical and also school psychologists, scientific, social workers, speech-language pathologists, learning professionals, as well as teachers, might each play an essential role in the ADHD assessment.

Similar to adults, there are no lab or imaging examinations available to make a medical diagnosis; instead, medical professionals base their verdicts on the evident signs and symptoms and also by dismissing other disorders. The expert that conducts your child's analysis will ask you a range of questions that you should address honestly and also freely. They may, additionally:

- Acquire a detailed clinical and also family history.
- Order or perform a necessary physical and neurological exam.
- Lead a thorough interview with you, your child, and your child's teacher(s).
- Uses of standardized testing tools for ADHD.
- Observe your child at play or school.

Getting your child reviewed for ADHD

Doctors, specialists, ADHD examinations – it might all feel a little frustrating to go for diagnosis for your child. You can take a lot of the turmoil out of the procedure with the following practical actions.

- Make an appointment with a professional.

As a parent, you can initiate testing for ADHD in support of your child. The earlier you arrange this consultation, the earlier you can get assist for their ADHD.

- Speak to your child's school.

Call your child's principal as well as speak directly as well as freely regarding your pursuit of a medical diagnosis. Public schools are needed by regulation to assist you, as well as in many cases, the staff wants to aid in enhancing your child's life at school.

- Give professionals the full understanding.

When you are asked the complicated concerns regarding your child's actions, be sure to address truthfully your viewpoint fundamental to the assessment procedure.

- Keep thing in check

You are your child's supporter, as well as have the power to stop hold-ups in getting a medical diagnosis. Check-in with physicians or professionals adequately and frequently to see where you are in the process.

If required, get a second opinion. If there is any type of uncertainty that your child has gotten a comprehensive or proper analysis, you can look for one more professional's help.

<u>Recognizing an ADHD diagnosis</u>

It's regular to feel upset or frightened by a diagnosis of ADHD. Yet keep in mind that getting a diagnosis can be the initial step towards making life better. As soon as you recognize what you're managing, you can begin getting treatment – which indicates taking control of signs and symptoms as well as feeling even more confident in every area of life.

An ADHD medical diagnosis might feel like a label. However, it might be extra valuable to consider it as an explanation. The diagnosis explains why you might have fought with life abilities such as paying attention, following directions, listening very carefully, organization – things that seem more normal to other individuals.

In this feeling, getting a medical diagnosis can be an alleviation. You can relax much more comfortable recognizing that it wasn't idleness or a lack of knowledge standing in your or your child's means, however rather a disorder that you can discover just how to handle.

Additionally, remember that an ADHD diagnosis is not a sentence for a lifetime of suffering. Some people have only mild signs and symptoms, while others experience even more pervasive issues. Despite where you or your child land on this range, there are many steps you can take to manage your signs and symptoms.

Co-existing problems and ADHD.

It is essential to recognize that an ADHD diagnosis does not dismiss other psychological health conditions. The following terms are not component of an ADHD diagnosis but sometimes co-occur with ADHD or get confused with it:

1. Anxiousness – Excessive fear that happens frequently and also is challenging to manage. Symptoms include feeling restless or on the side, quickly tired out, anxiety attack, irritability, muscle mass tension, and sleeping disorders.

2. Clinical depression –Symptoms consist of sensations of pessimism, helplessness, and also self-loathing, in addition to changes in sleep and too eating behaviors and even a loss of passion in activities you used to appreciate.

3. Learning impairment – Problems with comprehension, writing, or math. When

provided standardized tests, the trainee's capability or intelligence is considerably higher than their achievement.

4. Chemical abuse – The impulsivity and also behavioral issues that commonly accompany ADHD can lead to alcohol and even medication issues.

Getting help after an ADHD diagnosis

A medical diagnosis of ADHD can be an excellent wake-up call – it can provide you the added push you need to look for help for the signs and symptoms that are hindering your joy and success. If you or your child is detected with ADHD, don't wait to begin therapy. The earlier you start dealing with the symptoms, the better.

Taking care of ADHD is a job.

Discovering the right therapies for you or your child is a process— one that takes some time, perseverance, and also experimentation. But you can help yourself along the road by keeping the following goals in mind: discovering as much as you can around ADHD, getting a lot of support, and also adopting healthy and balanced lifestyle behaviors.

ADHD Is Treatable.

Don't surrender hope. With the right treatment and assistance, you or your child will certainly have the ability to get the signs of ADHD under control as well as develop the life that you desire.

Therapy is your very own responsibility.

It's up to you to do something about it to take care of the signs and symptoms of ADHD. Wellness specialists can help, but inevitably, the obligation lies in your very own hands.

Learning all you can around ADHD is vital.

Understanding the condition will assist you in making informed choices regarding all aspects of your or your child's life and also treatment.

Support makes all the difference.

While therapy depends on you, sustain from others can aid you to remain inspired as well as get you with bumpy rides.

GETTING GOING WITH YOUR ACTION PLAN

Organize the cooking area. Clean out the garage. Reach the fitness center. Send out thank you cards. Meal prep for the week. Pay the bill. ADHDers usually have lots they 'd like to obtain done, yet somehow their to-do lists never becomes any shorter. Why? Since merely deciding to do something isn't enough. You require an action strategy that consists of the "What, How, Where, When, Who", as well as "Why" for each task on your listing.

Preparation isn't something that comes naturally for many individuals with ADHD. That's because ADHDers commonly have weak executive feature abilities that regulate the capability to plan, arrange, and also handle their time successfully. Consequently, daily jobs may go by the wayside, or you might find yourself unprepared for those tasks you do begin as well as inevitably don't complete. Fortunately, with some preparation ahead of time, you'll be far better able to successfully tackle those to-do list items that never appear to get done.

Step 1: The What

When you prepare for any job, start with the end in mind: what EXACTLY are you attempting to achieve? What's your endgame? Exactly how will you know you've completed the job at hand? You require to recognize where you're going before you can plan on how you'll arrive.

Step 2: The How

How will I get this job done? Think about this action as your pre-plan. To simply put it: what factors need to be consisted of in your plan? Do you require materials? Do you need to work with the task at a specific time or in a particular area? Will you require help and additional details to get going? Are there multiple steps included? Exactly how will you manage interruptions and also various other possible obstructions?

Step 3: The Where

Where will you work on your task? This might seem like a no-brainer depending upon the activity; however, the area can be a crucial element when you have ADHD. You might need total silence with no disturbances to getthings done, or you might discover that you function well with a little bit of an ambient "buzz" around you and also are most productive functioning in your neighborhood coffee store. Even if you prepare to operate at home, you'll expect to consider the area: the kitchen table? Your work desk? On the couch in front of the TV?

Step 4: The When

Many individuals with ADHD deal with time monitoring, consisting of time ignorance, which implies you might have trouble accurately evaluating how much time something will take to complete. You may have additionally uncovered that if you do not set up or take a moment to do something, it doesn't get done. That's why "the When" is a necessary action in your planning. When do you prepare to do your task? When does it require to be completed? If there are numerous actions, what are the due dates for those? Be as precise as possible and set a pointer in either your planner or your phone, or you're sure to forget.

Tip 5: The Who

You'll want to think of what else requires to be a part of your plan. Take into consideration whether you'll need someone else's support with all or a component of your task. If you do, it'll be essential to collaborate with them, so they'll be proffered. You may likewise want to think about whether or not the job, at the very least in part, could be dealt with by another person, either in your family or an outside specialist.

Step 6: The Why

Last, however, absolutely not least, consider "the Why." When your inspiration to start or complete a product on your to-do list begins to wane, you'll intend to remember your "why." Why is completing this job vital to you? What do you want to get because of this? How will your life be simpler? How will you feel when it's done? Remembering your "why" will assist you in pressing through those "I don't feel like it" moments.

As the saying goes, "A goal without a strategy is just a desire." It takes more than merely deciding to do something to, in fact, get it done. In doing the task, use your time more effectively, as well as stay on track.

COPING WITH COMMON PROBLEMS IF YOU ARE A PARENT OF A CHILD WITH ADHD

Learn what you can do to supervise your child's habits and deal with common ADHD challenges.

How to aid your child with ADHD

Life with a child or teenager with attention deficit hyperactivity disorder (ADHD or ADD) can be aggravating, even overwhelming. As a parent you can aid your child to lessen daily challenges, direct their energy into favorable sectors, and also bring better tranquility to your household. Also, the earlier and a lot more consistently you address your child's troubles, the higher chance they have for success in life.

Children with ADHD usually have deficiencies in decision-making features: the ability to think and prepare in advance, organize, control impulses, and also complete tasks. That means you require to take over as the executive, providing added assistance while your child progressively acquires executive abilities of their own.

Although the signs and symptoms of ADHD can be absolutely nothing short of annoying, it's crucial to remember that the child who is neglecting, irritating, or awkward, is not acting willfully. Children with ADHD wish to sit silently; they intend to make their areas neat and also organized; they intend to do every little thing their parent says to do – but they don't know exactly how to make these things occur.

If you keep in mind that having ADHD is equally as discouraging for your child, it will be a great deal simpler to respond in favorable, supportive ways. With perseverance, empathy, and also lots of assistance, you can manage childhood years ADHD while taking pleasure in a steady, pleasing home.

ADHD and your family members

Before you can help effectively moms and dad a child with ADHD, it's vital to recognize the impact of your child's signs on the family members in its entirety. Children with ADHD exhibit a multitude of habits that can interfere with domesticity. They often do not "listen to" adult directions, so they do not obey them. They're disordered and also easily distracted, keeping another member of the family waiting. Or they start tasks as well as fail to remember to complete them – not to mention clean up after them. Children with impulsivity problems typically interrupt conversations, demand interest at inappropriate times, and talk before they assume, claiming thoughtless or embarrassing things. It's usually hard to get them to bed and also to sleep. Hyperactive children may damage things around your home and even put themselves in physical danger.

Due to these habits, brothers or sisters of children with ADHD deal with a variety of difficulties. Their needs commonly get much less attention than those of children with ADHD. They may be punished more severely when they err, as well as their successes maybe less renowned or considered less important. They may be enlisted as assistant parents – and condemned if the sibling with ADHD misbehaves under their supervision. Consequently, brothers or sisters may find their love for a brother or sister with ADHD mixed with envy and also resentment.

The need to monitor a child with ADHD can be physically and mentally exhausting. Your child's failure to "listen" can lead to aggravation and that aggravation to rage – adhered to by a sense of guilt concerning being angry at your child. Your child's behavior can make you nervous and worried. If there's a fundamental difference between your personality that of your child with ADHD, their behavior can be particularly challenging to accept.

To satisfy the challenges of raising a child with ADHD, you should be able to master a mix of concern and uniformity. Staying in a house that gives both loves as well as the structure is the very best point for a child or teenager who is discovering to manage ADHD.

ADHD parenting suggestion 1:

Stay positive as well as healthy yourself

As a mom and dad, you set the stage for your child's psychological and physical health and wellness. You have control over most of the factors that can positively influence the signs of your child's problem.

Keep a positive attitude. Your most beautiful properties for assisting your child in satisfying the challenges of ADHD are your positive mindset as well as sound judgment. When you are calm and concentrated, you are much more likely to be able to connect with your child, assisting him or her to be tranquil as well as focused.

Keep things in perspective. Keep in mind that your child's behavior is related to a disorder. A lot of the time, it is not intentional. Hold on to your sense of humor. What's awkward today might be a fun family member's tale ten years from now.

Don't sweat the tiny things and make some compromises. One task left undone isn't a massive deal when your child has finished two others plus the day's work. If you are a nit-picker, you will not just be dissatisfied continuously but also create impossible assumptions for your child with ADHD.

Rely on your child. Think of or make a written checklist of whatever that declares, significant, as well as distinct regarding your child. Based on that: your child can discover, change, mature, and be successful. Declare this every day as you clean your teeth or make your coffee.

Self-care

As your child's good example and also an essential resource of strength, it is crucial that you live a healthy life. If you are overtired or lack patience, you run the risk of losing sight of the framework and assistance you have so carefully set up for your child with ADHD.

Seek assistance

Among one of the most vital things to keep in mind in rearing a child with ADHD is that you do not have to do it alone. Speak with your child's physicians, specialists, and instructors. Join an orderly support system for moms and dads of children with ADHD. These groups supply an online forum for providing as well as getting advice and give a safe place to air vent feelings as well as share experiences.

Take breaks.

Friends and family members can be great choices to use to babysit, but you may feel guilty about leaving your child or leaving the volunteer with a child with ADHD. Next time, approve their offer and also talk about exactly how ideal it is to manage your child.

Take care of yourself.

Eat right, workout, and discover ways to decrease stress and anxiety, whether it suggests taking a nighttime bath or practicing early morning meditation. If you do get ill, recognize it as well as get assistance.

ADHD Parenting Suggestion 2:

Establish structure and also adhere to it

Children with ADHD are most likely to succeed in finishing tasks when the tasks happen in foreseeable patterns and foreseeable places. Your work is to produce and suffer structure in your house to ensure that your child understands what to anticipate as well as what they are expected to do.

Tips for assisting your child with ADHD to keep focused and also organized:

1. Follow a regimen.

It is essential to establish a time and an area for every little thing to assist the child with ADHD to comprehend as well as meet assumptions. Develop basic and also predictable routines for dishes, homework, play, as well as sleep time. Have your child set out garments for the following early morning before going to bed, and also make sure whatever she or he needs to take to school is in a unique place, where they are easy to get a hold of.

2. Use clocks and timers.

Consider placing clocks all through the house, with a large one in your child's room. Permit enough time for what your child requires to do, such as studying or getting ready in the early morning. Make use of a timer for homework or transitional times, such as in between finishing up play as well as preparing for bed.

Streamline your child's schedule. It is excellent to stay clear of quiet time, but a child with ADHD may end up being much more distracted and "end up" if there are lots of after-school tasks. You might require to make adjustments to the child's after-school commitments based on the individual child's capacities and also the needs of particular activities.

3. Create a peaceful area.

Make sure your child has a quiet, private room of their very own. A surface or a bedroom area is suitable, as long as it's not the same place as the child goes for a break.

Do your best to be neat and also arranged. Set up your residence in an orderly way. Make sure your child understands that every little thing has its place. Lead by example with neatness and organization as much as possible.

4. Stay clear of troubles by keeping children with ADHD occupied!

For children with ADHD, still, time might intensify their signs and also create chaos in your house. It is essential to maintain a child with ADHD busy without overdoing a lot of things that the child ends up being overwhelmed.

Sign your child up for a sport, art class, or music. In your home, arrange straightforward tasks that fill your child's time. These can be tasks like aiding you to prepare, playing a board game with a sibling, or drawing. Try not to over-rely on the television or computer/video games as time-fillers. However, TV and also video games are increasingly violent and also may only enhance your child's signs of ADHD.

ADHA parenting suggestion 3:

Encourage movement as well as rest

Children with ADHD commonly have the power to shed. Organized sports and various other exercises can assist them in getting their energy out in healthy and balanced means and concentrate their interest in specific activities as well as abilities. The advantages of training are unlimited: it boosts focus, reduces depression as well as anxiousness, and promotes mental development. Most importantly, for children with attention deficiencies, however, is the reality that exercise leads to far better sleep, which in turn can also lower the signs and symptoms of ADHD.

Find a sporting activity that your child will enjoy, and that fits their stamina. For example, sporting activities such as softball that involve a lot of "downtime" are not the very best suitable for children with ADHD. Individual or group sporting activities like basketball and hockey that call for constant movement are better options. Children with ADHD might likewise take advantage of training in martial arts (such as tae kwon do) or yoga exercise, which boosts mental control as they work out the body.

Not enough rest can make any person less conscientious, yet it can be extremely destructive for children with ADHD. Children with ADHD need at least as much rest as their untouched peers but often tend not to get what they need. Their interest problems can result in overstimulation as well as problems sleeping. A constant, very early bedtime is one of the most practical strategies to battle this issue. However, it might not fix it.

Assist your child to improve rest by checking out one or more of the following strategies:

1. Decrease tv time and also enhance your child's activities and exercise degrees during the day.

2. Eliminate Caffeine From Your Child's Diet.
3. Produce a buffer time to decrease the task level for an hour or two before bedtime. Locate quieter activities such as coloring, reviewing, or playing quietly.
4. Spend 10 mins cuddling with your child. It will build a sense of love as well as protection as well as give time to cool down.
5. Usage lavender or other aromas in your child's room. The scent may aid in relaxing your child.
6. Use leisure tapes as recorded sound for your child when falling asleep. There are several ranges available consisting of nature audios and calming songs. Children with ADHD commonly find "white noise" to be relaxing. You can develop white sound by placing a radio on fixed or running an electric fan.

The advantages of "green time" in children with hyperactivity

Research shows that children with ADHD gain from hanging out in nature. Children experience a better decrease in signs and symptoms of ADHD when they play in a park loaded with the yard and also trees than on a concrete play area. Bear in mind of this promising as well as a primary method for managing ADHD. Even in cities, many family members have access to parks as well as various other all-natural setups. Join your children in this "eco-friendly time" – you'll additionally obtain a much-deserved breath of fresh air for yourself.

ADHD Parenting Suggestion 4:

Set Clear Expectations And Rules

Children with ADHD need consistent policies that they can understand as well as comply with. Make the rules of actions for the family simple and clear. Jot down the guidelines and hang them up in an area where your child can easily read them.

Children with ADHD react particularly well to arranged systems of incentives as well as effects. It's essential to describe what will occur when the regulations are complied with as well as when they are damaged. Stick to your system: comply with through each as well as every time with an incentive or a consequence.

As you develop these permanent structures, remember that children with ADHD usually obtain objection. Watch permanently actions – as well as praise it. Praise is especially crucial for children that have ADHD because they typically get so little of it. These children receive an adjustment, remediation, and grievances concerning their behavior – but little favorable reinforcement.

A smile, favorable comment, or various other benefits from you can improve the attention, focus as well as impulse control of your child with ADHD. Do your best to focus on giving positive praise for proper behavior as well as job completion, while providing as few adverse responses as feasible to unsuitable habits or inadequate job efficiency. Compensate your child for small successes that you could take for granted in one more child.

Making Use Of Rewards as well as Consequences

Incentives

- Reward your child with benefits, appreciation, or activities, rather than with food or toys.
- Change awards frequently. Children with ADHD obtain bored if the benefit is always the same.
- Make a chart with things or stars awarded for the right actions, so your child has a beautiful reminder of their successes.
- Immediate rewards function far better than the pledge of a future reward, however

small benefits causing a huge one can likewise function.

– Always follow through with an incentive.

Consequences

– Consequences must be defined in advance and take place right away after your child has misbehaved.
– Try breaks as well as the elimination of benefits as repercussions for misbehavior.
– Remove your child from situations as well as environments that activate unacceptable habits.
– When your child is mischievous, ask what she or he could have done instead. After that, have your child show it.
– Always follow through with a consequence.

ADHD Parenting Suggestion 5:

Help your child consume right

Diet is not a straight root cause of attention shortage condition, yet food can and does influence your child's psychological state, which in turn seems to affect actions. Monitoring and also changing what, when, and also how much your child eats can help reduce the signs of ADHD.

All children take advantage of fresh foods, routine mealtimes, and also staying away from fast food. These tenets are especially real for children with ADHD, whose spontaneity and distractedness can result in missed out on dishes, disordered eating, as well as over-eating.

Children with ADHD are infamous for not eating regularly. Without parental guidance, these children could not eat for hours and afterward binge on whatever is about. The result of this pattern can be ruining the child's physical and also psychological wellness.

Prevent harmful consuming practices by scheduling regular nourishing meals or snacks for your child no more than three hours apart. Physically, a child with ADHD needs a constant intake of healthy and balanced food; emotionally, mealtimes are a required break and a setup rhythm to the day.

- Do away with the junk foods in your home.
- Place fatty and also sweet foods off-limits when eating in restaurants.
- Switch off tv shows riddled with junk-food ads.
- Give your child an everyday vitamin-and-mineral supplement.

ADHD Parenting Suggestion 6:

Teach your child just how to make friends

Children with ADHD typically have a problem with necessary social communications. They might battle with reading social cues, talk way too much, disturb regularly, or come off as hostile or "also extreme." Their psychological immaturity can make them stand apart among children their very own age, as well as make them targets for hostile teasing.

Do not forget, though, that lots of children with ADHD are incredibly smart and imaginative as well as will at some point figure out for themselves how to get along with others and avoid people who aren't suitable as good friends. Character traits that could annoy parents and also educators may come throughout to peers as amusing and fun.

Helping a child with ADHD boost social abilities

It's tough for children with ADHD to discover social skills as well as social rules. You can aid your child with ADHD to become a far better listener, learn to review individuals' faces as well as body language, and also engage even more efficiently in teams.

Speak delicately, however, honestly with your child concerning their difficulties as well as just how to make modifications.Role-play different social scenarios with your child; Trade frequently functions as well as attempts to make it enjoyable.

Beware to select friends for your child with comparable language as well as physical skills.Welcome only one or two friends at once in the beginning. See them carefully while they play and also have a zero-tolerance policy for hitting, pushing as well as screaming.

Make time as well as an area for your child to play, and also compensate for significant play behaviors commonly.

DISCIPLINE, COMMUNICATION AND THE ADHD CHILD

Parenting Dos and Don'ts: ADHD and Discipline

Do: Shift Your Mindset

With ADHD, typical methods of the technique aren't always the most effective fit. Shift your attitude from "I need to self-control my child" and also get interested in how to aid them to boost their skills. Taking a mindset of, "What can I do to aid them" instead of "How can I obtain them to do what I desire" is a game-changer.

Do: Ask Yourself This Question

Are your child's habits mischievous? Put, is he purposefully making a poor selection, or dealing with the impulsivity that usually comes with ADHD? A lot of children that have ADHD understand what they must do but cannot get themselves to do it. If you select to see it as something they wish to do, however, is having a hard time with, you're more likely to lead favorably rather than punish.

Do not: Yell

If your little girl gets sidetracked and also really did not do her homework, take a deep breath. If you yell, it will not alter anything. She'll close down and also not listen to anything you state. Even if it does seem to "work" in the short-term, it's harmful because your child is just motivated by worry. You desire your child to trust you. Don't project what it looks like to lose control.

Do: Be Brief

When you communicate with a child that has ADHD, obtain his attention. Keep it brief and also comfortable. If you make a demand, ensure he recognizes it. If it's a high demand – It's time to speak about your grades, for instance – have the conversation over a collection of days or weeks. It gives him time to process.

Do not: Think Too Far Ahead

Even if your child does not finish tidying up his unpleasant space today doesn't indicate he'll never see thingsthrough. You do not need to have your child master every little thing today. With your support as well as assistance, he'll discover each ability when he's ready. Construct your method to the future rather than worrying about what it could look like.

Do: Learn and also Be Compassionate

You cannot see the internal functions of your child's brain. All you see is your child's habits. That can be frustrating as well as complicated. Much like in any other attempting situation, it assists in being educated and understanding. Check out all you can around ADHD from relied on resources, so you recognize the problem, and also be compassionate with your child as well as on yourself.

Don't: Ask Too Much of Your Child

Children with ADHD cannot regulate themselves in the same way as other children the very same age. They may do something well one day and also not do it well the next. It's way too much to ask a child with ADHD to be consistent. You'll both feel a lot better if you praise your child where she or he rests in any provided moment.

Do: Celebrate the Wins

Take notice of what goes well. Maybe your child increased his qualities or he still leaves all the lights on in your home. Change your perspective so that you see as well as commemorate what worked out. Reinforce the good as opposed to just dwelling on what you 'd like to be different. When your child does what they understand well, highlight the initiative, and also what caused the actions. "You got your homework done. You need to feel so pleased with doing it yourself. How did that take place so we can keep this going?"

Do not: Address Every Little Thing

Children with ADHD are wrong often. They get redirected throughout the day, daily. If you take on everything regularly, it'll tire you both out. Select one or two habits to deal with and let the remainder stay for now. You'll reach them at some point. This way, your child won't have that "I can't do anything best" feeling regularly.

Do: Coach and also Collaborate

You wouldn't anticipate your child to comprehend precisely how to play football without an instructor. You likewise cannot expect them to manage themselves when their brains aren't wired to inform them exactly how. Train as well as collaborate with your child so that they can practice abilities as well as decision-making in a risk-free environment. Exercise with expressions like, "How do you assume we should manage this scenario?" Listen and afterward determine what's most beautiful.

Do: Look for the Opportunities

Your child cannot sit still at supper. She continues popping up and running about. However, she's been handling her behavior at school throughout the day and also is tired. Change your expectations, so she does not feel pity for making mistakes. Set an objective for her to settle down for merely two mins. Or select it and let her be the person that gets the ketchup and removes plates from the table.

Do: Punish Every Child Fairly

If you have more than one child and they do not all have ADHD, their consequences many be different. That can be a complicated region for moms and dads. Tell all your children that you're a team, and also consequences will undoubtedly be reasonable; however, not regularly the same. Show concern when any one of your children feels upset. Say, "I recognize this might be hard for you to accept."

Do: Take Care of Yourself

ADHD actions can be tough to deal with. When you're tranquil as well as rested, you can deal with more and also handle it better. It may suggest you cut down on dedications and readjust your timetable and standards. Self-care – like exercise, rest, and a great diet regimen – is additionally vital. This way, you're better organized to help your household – as well as yourself – flourish.

HANDLING HOMEWORK FOR A CHILD WITH ADHD

Launching your child for success at school

The classroom setting can present obstacles for a child with attention deficit disorder (ADHD or ADD). The actual tasks these learners find the hardest – staying still, paying attention quietly, focusing – are the ones they are called for to do all day long. Maybe most frustrating of all is that most of these children want to have the ability to discover and behave like their untouched peers. Neurological deficits, not hesitation, keep children with attention deficit disorder from discovering in conventional means.

As a parent, you can help your child to deal with these deficits and also conquer the difficulties schooling develops. You can work with your child to put into action practical approaches for discovering both in and out of the classroom as well as connect with teachers about just how your child learns best. With regular support, the following strategies can aid your child joy in discovering, overcome instructional challenges – and experience success at school and also past.

Tips for working with educators

Remember that your child's educator has a full plate: along with taking care of a group of children with unique individualities as well as learning styles, they can likewise expect to have at the very least one student with ADHD. Teachers might try their best to assist your child with a ADHD in learning, however, parental participation can substantially boost your child's education. You have the power to maximize your child's possibilities for success by supporting the actions absorbed in the class. If you can work with and also help your child's educator, you can directly affect the knowledge of your child with ADHD at school.

There are several ways you can collaborate with instructors to keep your child on a course at school. With each other, you can assist your child with ADHD in learning how to find their feet in the classroom and also work successfully through the challenges of the school day. As a parent, you are your child's supporter. For your child to do well in the classroom, you must connect their demands to the adults at school. It is equally vital for you to listen to what the educators and also various other school officials have to state.

You can ensure that interaction with your child'sschool is useful as well as practical. Try to keep in mind that your joint function is figuring out how to best assist your childin being successful in school. Whether you talk over the phone, email, or meet personally, make an initiative to be calm, detailed, and, most importantly, positive – a unique perspective can go a long way when communicating with school.

Tip 1: Plan in advance.

You can prepare to consult with school officials or instructors before the school year even starts. If the year has begun, plan to talk with a teacher or therapist on at least a month-to-month basis.

Have meetings. Settle on a time that benefits both you as well as your child's teacher and adhere to it. If it's hassle-free, meet in your child's classroom so you can get a feeling of your child's physical learning setting.

Tip 2: Produce goals with each other.

Discuss your hopes for your child's school's success. With each other, make a note of individual as well as practical objectives as well as speak about exactly how to help your child reach them.

Tip 3: Listen thoroughly.

Like you, your child's teacher wants to see your child be successful at school. Listen to what they have to say – even if it is sometimes difficult to listen to. Understanding your child's obstacles in school is crucial to discovering remedies that work.

Tip 5: Share information.

You recognize your child's history, as well as your child's instructor sees them daily. With each other, you have a lot of details that can result in a far better understanding of your child's difficulties. Share your observations easily, as well as motivate your child's instructors to do the same.

Tip 6: Ask the hard questions and offer a complete picture.

Make sure to specify any medicines your child takes and describe any other therapies. Share with your child's instructor which methods work well – and also which do not – for your child in the house. Ask if your child is having any troubles in school, including on the playground. Learn if your child is qualified for any special services to help with knowing.

Tip 7: Creating as well as using a behavior plan

Children with ADD/ADHD can influence proper classroom behavior. However, they need structure and clear expectations to keep their signs and symptoms in check. As a parent, you can assist by developing a routine prepare for your child – and also following it. Whatever sort of behavior plan you decide to execute, develop it in close collaboration with your child's instructor as well as your child.

Children with an attention problem respond best to details goals and also everyday positive reinforcement – as well as valuable benefits. Yes, you may have to hang a carrot on a stick with inspiring your child to act much better in the course. Produce a plan that includes small incentives for small success and more significant benefits for more massive accomplishments.

Tips for managing ADHD symptoms at school

ADHD impacts each child's mind in different ways so that each instance can look entirely various in the classroom. Children with ADHD exhibit a variety of signs and symptoms: some seem to bounce around, some dream frequently, and also others cannot appear to follow the guidelines.

As a parent, you can assist your child with ADHD to reduce any type of or every one of these sorts of actions. It is essential to comprehend just how attentiondeficit disorder impacts different children's activities so that you can select the proper methods for dealing with the problem. There is a range of relatively uncomplicated approaches you and your child's teacher can require to most effectively take care of the signs of ADHD – and make your child's journey in school a success.

Handling distractibility

Students with ADHD might end up being so quickly distracted by noises, passersby, or their thoughts that they frequently miss out on vital class details. These children have difficulty staying focused on tasks that call for sustained mental effort. They may seem as if they're listening to you, yet something gets in the way of their capacity to preserve the details.

Assisting children who sidetrack easily includes physical positioning, increased movement, and also breaking long stretches of learning into much shorter chunks.

Seat the child with ADHD away from windows and doors. Put family pets in another room or outside while the student is working.

Alternative seated activities with will enable the child to move their body around the space whenever feasible, so integrate physical movement directly into lessons.

Write vital information down where the child can conveniently review and review it. Remind the pupil where the data is located.

Split massive projects into smaller ones, and also enable constant breaks.

Reducing interrupting

Children with ADHD might struggle with managing their impulses, so they typically speak up of turn. In the class, they call out or comment while others are speaking. Their outbursts may encounter as aggressive and even rude, creating social troubles as well. The self-esteem of children with ADHD is frequently reasonably fragile, so dealing with this concern publicly in class or before family members doesn't help the issue – and also may even make problems worse.

Fixing the disruptions of children with ADHD must be done very carefully so that the child's self-worth is preserved, particularly before others. Establish a "secret language" with the child with ADHD. You can use discreet gestures or words you have formerly agreed upon to allow the child to know they are disrupting. Praise the child for interruption-free discussions.

Managing impulsivity

Children with ADHD may act before thinking, developing challenging social situations, along with problems in the classroom. Children who have difficulty with impulse control might come off as aggressive or unruly. This is probably the most turbulent symptom of ADHD, specifically at school.

Techniques for handling impulsivity consist of behavior plans, the prompt method for infractions, and a procedure for offering children with ADHD a feeling of control over their day.

Make sure a written behavior plan is near the trainee. You can also tape it to the wall surface or the child's work desk.

Give consequences instantly, complying with wrongdoing. Specify in your description, making sure the child recognizes how they misbehaved.

Identify good behavior out loud. Be specific in your appreciation, seeing to it the child knows what they did right.

Compose the routine for the day on the board or on a paper as well as cross off each thing as it is finished. Children with ADHD might acquire a sense of control and feel calmer when they recognize what to anticipate.

Handling fidgeting as well as attention deficit disorder

Students with ADHD experience the impulse for frequent, constant physical movement. It might appear like a battle for these children to stay in their seats. Children with ADD/ADHD might leap, kick, twist, fidget as well as move – ways that make them difficult to teach.

Strategies for combating hyperactivity include creative means to allow the child with ADHD to move in proper ways at proper times. Releasing energy in this manner may make it much easier for the child to keep their bodies calmer during work time.

Ask children with ADHD to run a duty or complete a task for you, even if it just suggests strolling across the room to collect pencils or place meals away.

Urge a child with ADHD to play a sporting activity – or a minimum of run about before and after school – and also make sure the child never misses out on recess or P.E.

Provide a tension round, tiny toy, or one more item for the child to squeeze or play with discreetly at their seat.

Restrict screen time in favor of time for physical activities.

Managing difficulty following directions

Difficulty following instructions is a hallmark issue for numerous children with ADHD. These children might resemble they understand as well as may even make a note of trends, yet after that aren't able to follow them as asked. In some cases, these learners miss-steps as well as turn in an insufficient job or misconstrue a task altogether and also wind up doing another thing entirely.

Helping children with ADHD comply with directions means taking steps to break down and reinforce the steps associated with your guidelines, and also redirecting when essential. Try keeping your activities simple, allowing the child to complete one action and, after that, return to discover what they ought to do next. If the child leaves the path, provide a tranquil suggestion, redirecting in a calm yet firm voice. Whenever possible, compose instructions down in a bold pen or colored chalk on a blackboard.

Tips for making learning fun

One positive way to maintain your child's interest concentrated on learning is to make the process enjoyable. Using physical activity in a lesson, attaching dull facts to fascinating trivia, or developing silly songs that make information much more comfortable to remember can aid your child delight in learning and even decrease the symptoms of ADHD.

Assisting children with ADHD delight in math

Children who have an ADHD tend to think in a "concrete" fashion. They naturally desire to hold, touch, or take part in experience to learn something brand-new. By utilizing video games as well as objects to show mathematical concepts, you can reveal your child that math can be purposeful – and also fun.

Play video games.

Use flash memory cards, dice, or dominoes to make numbers fun. Or merely utilize your fingers and toes, putting them in or shaking them when you add or deduct.

Attract pictures.

Specifically, for word troubles, illustrations can help children better recognize mathematical principles. If words problem claims, there are twelve cars, help your child draw them from the guiding wheel to the trunk.

Create foolish acronyms. To bear in mind the order of operations, as an example, make up a track or expression that uses the initial letter of each procedure in the proper order.

Helping children with ADHD enjoy reading

There are numerous means to make reading amazing, even if the skill itself often tends to present a battle for children with ADHD. Bear in mind that analysis at its a lot of fundamental level includes stories and interesting details – which all children delight in.

Read to children. Make this activity a relaxing, quality time with you.

Make predictions or "bets." Frequently ask the child what they assume could occur next. Design prediction: "The lady in the story seems rather hands on – I bet she's most likely to try to conserve her household."

Act out the story. Let the child select their character and also designate you one. Use funny voices as well as outfits to bring it to life.

Exactly how does your child like to learn?

When children are given information in such a way that makes it very easy for them to absorb, learning is a lot of extra fun. If you recognize just how your child with ADHD learns best, you can develop delightful lessons that pack an informational punch.

Auditory learners learn best by talking as well as listening. Have these children recite facts to a favored track. Let them pretend they get on a radio show and also deal with others typically.

Visual students learn best with testing or watching. Let them enjoy with various fonts on the computer system and also use tinted flashcards to examine. Enable them to write or draw their ideas theoretically.

Kinesthetic learners learn best through physical touch or movement as part of a lesson. For these learners, provide jellybeans for counters as well as outfits for acting out components of literature or history. Allow them to make use of clay and make collections.

Tips for understanding homework

Certain, children might globally dread it – however, for moms and dad of a child with ADHD, homework is a gold possibility. Academic work done outside the class offers you as the moms and dad with an opportunity to successfully nurture your child. It's time you can help your child prosper at school where you both feel most comfortable: your living-room.

With your support, children with ADHD can utilize research time not just for mathematics troubles or creating essays, but additionally for practicing the administrative and also research study skills they require to flourish in the class.

Aiding a child with ADHD being organized

When it pertains to the school, it can assist in getting a fresh start. Also, if it's not the begin of the school year, go patronize your child and select school products that include folders, a three-ring binder, and also color-coded dividers. Assist the child to place their papers right into this brand-new arrangement.

Establish a research folder for finished research and also arrange loose papers by color-coding folders. Show your child how to file suitably.

Aid your child to organize their belongings every day, including knapsack, folders, as well as even pockets.

If possible, maintain an additional set of textbooks as well as various other materials in the house.

Assist your child in discovering to make as well as use checklists, crossing products off as they accomplish them.

Assisting a child with ADHD obtain homework done on time

Recognizing concepts as well as being organized are two activities in the right direction. Still, homework also has to be completed in a single evening – and finished on time. Help a child with ADHD to the finish line with techniques that supply constant structure.

Select a particular time and area for research that is as free as possible of clutter, family pets, as well as a TV.

Enable the child breaks as typically as every 10 to 20 minutes.

Educate a far better understanding of the passage of time: use an analog clock as well as timers to monitor homework efficiency.

Establish a homework procedure at school: develop a place where the pupil can quickly discover their finished homework and also select a consistent time to hand in work to the teacher.

Other means to aid your child with homework

Encourage workout as well as sleep. Physical activity improves focus as well as promotes mind development. Significantly for children with ADHD, it also leads to better rest, which consequently can decrease the ADHD signs and symptoms.

Help your child eat. Setting up regular healthy dishes and snacks while cutting back on junk and sugary foods can assist manage signs and symptoms of ADHD.

Deal with yourself, so you're far better able to take care of your child. Do not disregard your needs. Try to consume right, exercise, get sufficient rest, handle stress, and seek in-person assistance from family and friends.

TRIGGER FOODS FOR ADHD

Managing ADHD: 15 Foods to Avoid

ADHD, additionally known as Attention Deficit Hyperactivity Disorder, is a type of behavioral problem mostly seen in children. This disorder is identified by restlessness, inattentiveness, difficulty focusing, high degrees of indistinct energy, and impulsive actions. While a correct diet plan cannot heal ADHD, people that follow specific dietary standards can benefit from eating effectively.

ADHD Medications

Many professionals think consuming certain foods can cause ADHD symptoms in individuals, particularly children, so it's important to avoid specific foods thought to stimulate a reaction.

If you or a person you love struggles with ADHD, try avoiding these 15 foods. Getting rid of (or firmly reducing) these foods from your diet can assist handle the symptoms of ADHD.

1. Ice Cream

Dairy items, such as ice cream, can set off ADHD in individuals that are oversensitive to milk items. Somebody who is sensitive to dairy items might feel weary, both as well as psychologically, after eating foods such as gelato. Because of this, it's best to avoid this chilly reward – although it may seem like a great concept at the time.

2. Yogurt

Similar to ice cream, yogurt is a milk item that has been known to stimulate flare-ups in individuals with ADHD. Removing these types of products (milk items) entirely from your diet for a couple of weeks will undoubtedly assist youin seeing whether they are a cause for ADHD. If dairy items activate your ADHD, think about changing them for foods made with soy instead.

3. Sugar

Professionals say a diet high in sugar can stimulate a flare in ADHD patients. Numerous experts think that the sugar strips your body of the vitamins, enzymes, and also minerals called for to support your mood.

4. Coffee

This might be a difficult one for numerous people to surrender, considering coffee is such a popular beverage. Lots of people count on coffee for an energetic start to their mornings. However, coffee contains a substantial quantity of high levels of caffeine, which – an all-natural energizer understood to activate ADHD symptoms. If your symptoms get worse after drinking coffee, you can try drinking herbal teas or decaffeinated coffee instead.

5. Swordfish

Fish high in mercury, such as swordfish, have been recognized to cause ADHD signs and symptoms. The heavy metal (mercury) discovered in this type of fish can reduce one's capability to concentrate and also hinder focus in many individuals. If you discover your symptoms getting worse after eating this type of fish, select fish with reduced mercury levels such as shrimp, lobster or salmon.

6. Cheese

One more dairy food to stay clear of when attempting to prevent stimulating ADHD signs is cheese (especially cow's cheese). Similar to yogurt and ice cream, getting rid of cheese from your diet plan for six to eight weeks will assist in determining whether it's the cause for your flare-ups. If you observe your symptoms are extra manageable when you're not eating cheese (or various other cow dairy items), think about switching over to a lactose-free or cow dairy products free diet (i.e., eat goat's cheese rather).

7. Chocolate

Chocolate, like coffee, consists of a significant amount of caffeine. High levels of caffeine have been known to trigger ADHD signs and also can make signs even worse if you select not to eliminate it from your diet plan. If you notice, your symptoms worsen after consuming chocolate then reduce intake.

8. Pop/Soda

Pop has human-made colors and flavoring, which several experts think can trigger signs in individuals with ADHD. In addition to human-made colors and flavor, numerous brands also have higher degrees of caffeine, which – as explained formerly – can activate ADHD signs and symptoms also. It's finest to avoid soda and go with a natural drink (homemade smoothies are incredible) instead.

9. Frozen Pizza

Icy pizzas are stuffed packed with synthetic shades as well as flavors, much like pop. The ingredients utilized to help enhance these types of products can raise attention deficit disorder and also decrease concentration in individuals with this condition. If you like consuming pizza, take into consideration making one from scratchyourself. In this manner, you'll know every one of the active ingredients made use of are healthy and balanced and also natural

10. Corn

Yellow vegetables, such as corn, are known to trigger responses in people with ADHD. It is suggested that you avoid eating these types of veggies to help regulate your signs and symptoms. If you wish to eat healthily, opt for various other vegetables like spinach, peppers or tomatoes

11. Chips

It's virtually a known fact that chips would be on this list. A lot of fast food must be prevented tohandle this type of problem. Chips are also high in artificial colors as well as flavoring, makes them a poor choice for individuals trying to find an ADHD bland diet. If you like snacking, take into consideration consuming healthy and balanced vegetables to suppress your cravings, instead of fast food like chips and delicious chocolate.

12. Squash

Squash is one more yellow food to avoid when managing ADHD. For the same factors as corn, squash has been recognized to create flare-ups. Not all yellow foods misbehave for people with ADHD – bananas are all right since the real banana is white. Only the peel of the bananas is yellow, as well as you don't eat the yellow component anyways. As we pointed out earlier, select other healthy (perhaps natural) veggies instead of yellow ones.

13. Fruit Juice

Many fruit juices are loaded with artificial colors and flavors. You need to avoid consuming fruit juices unless they are 100 percent natural without artificial coloring or flavor. Consider making a delicious healthy smoothie with fresh, organic fruits you've bought from the grocery store as opposed to boxed juice that's undesirable for several factors.

14. Junk food

Fast Food gets on the top of most "Do Not Eat" checklists, and this list is no exception. The fried foods found in the majority of fast food dishes are unbelievably unhealthy, and the active ingredients have been recognized to cause an increase in

ADHD symptoms. People seeking to handle their signs and symptoms need to stay clear of fast food entirely as well as select making dinner yourself.

15. Red Meat

Red meat has been understood to create an increase of symptoms for ADHD patients, experts state. Reducing your red meat intake (not necessarily eradicating it) may verify terrific benefits when it comes to controlling your ADHD. As pointed out previously, going with much healthier choices like salmon or shrimp will undoubtedly aid in keeping your symptoms managed so you can maintain a more active, better life.

THE IMPORTANCE OF KEEPING AN ADHD JOURNAL

Coping with a mental wellness problem can be difficult, yet journaling might aid. Journaling can help you to handle anxiety, anxiousness, depression, and also bipolar illness. Also, you can utilize your journal to assist you in improving your routines as well as behaviors. To begin journaling, select a convenient time to write each day as well as allow yourself to write whatever involves your mind for 20 minutes. Utilize your journal to process your feelings or deal with your self-improvement goals.

Determine if you intend to maintain a paper journal or an electronic journal.

Usually, writing by hand aids – you refine your ideas much better. Nonetheless, it's ideal to choose whichever style is most convenient for you. Choose a paper journal if you delight in composing by handor utilize a word processor if you prefer to type.

A paper journal will make it less complicated to get imaginative with your entries if you're interested in including art in your journal.

You may be able to include in your digital journal from any device if you use Google Docs. Download Google Docs free of charge from the app store. After that, produce as well as modify records on any device that has Google Docs.

Write in your journal daily to get one of the most benefits.

It's essential to create a practice if you intend to use your journal to boost your mental wellness. Pick a time when it's convenient for you to write; after that, challenge yourself to create daily. Arrange your journaling time right into your day like any various other essential discussion.

You might compose in your journal every early morning when you wake up, during your lunch hour, or directly before bed.

If you commute by bus or train, use that time to write in your journal.

Set a timer for 20 minutes as well as attempt to create until it goes off.

When you first start journaling, provide yourself a brief home window of time to do it, so it does not feel overwhelming. Begin with 20 mins, but feel free to readjust the time to fit your requirements better. While the timer is going, write down or type any words that stand out into your head.

While the goal is to discuss your thoughts or stress factors, do not bother with that right now. It's all right to compose things like, "I don't understand what to claim," "This feels silly," or "I can't think of anything today." If you keep going, you'll begin to discover your internal thoughts.

Pointer: it's okay to keep creating after the timer goes off. The objective of the timer is to assist you in feeling like there's a structure to your journaling practice, which may help you start much more conveniently.

Don't bother with punctuation or grammar.

Your journal is for you, so it doesn't matter if you make use of appropriate sentences or spell words appropriately. Let your thoughts circulation openly with no self-editing.

If your grammar mistakes honestly bother you, it's alright to return and correct them at a later time. Nevertheless, this isn't needed.

Get creative with your formatting if you do not know, such as writing in sentences.

You can still get the benefits of journaling even if you hate writing or can't determine what to state. Don't bother with having sentences or paragraphs. Try various ways of formatting entrances until you find one that works for you. Below are some ways you might express yourself:

- Make a list.
- Create a rhyme or song.
- Include photos to reveal precisely how you feel or what's on your mind.
- Write a letter to somebody.
- Create a tale with you as a significant personality.
- Use sentence stems from your specialist or online. These could include, "I feel most dismayed when ...," "I feel my ideal when ... " or "I'm most anxious concerning ...".
- Make A Bullet Journal

Make Your Journal A Judgment-Free Zone

Provide on your approval to compose whatever you're feeling without policing your ideas. Do not attach negative emotions like regret or shame to what you write. You have every right to your thoughts and also feelings, and your journaling technique is your way that helps you be as healthy and balanced as possible. Do not judge yourself for making this excellent step towards fixing your internal problems.

You may feel guilty for raving out over something that took place in your day. Do not judge yourself for getting distressed since that's an entirely reasonable reaction. Instead, pat yourself on the back for working through those ideas in your journal.

Managing Thoughts and also Feelings

Express whatever is on your mind when you sit down to write.

The most effective means to use journaling to refine your ideas and feelings is to blog about what's going on in your life that day. Discuss what's happened to you, how you feel about things, as well as any worries that you have. Keep writing until your timer goes off, or you feel much better.

You might create something like, "Today, I felt awkward since it was drizzling all the time. I assume the weather condition influences my state of mind. I question how I can help myself feel better on gloomy days."

Write in a stream of thoughts when you're not sure what you're feeling.

Occasionally it's tough to understand what's really on your mind, which's fine! To create a stream of aware, take-down any words that enter your account, even if they don't make good sense. Don't worry about spelling or syntax. Keep creating up until you recognize a central point or motif arising, which will certainly inform of you exactly how you feel.

As an example, a stream of mindful entrance might resemble this: "Sitting right here simply not recognizing what to state it's been a long day as well as I'm exhausted, but I can't identify why I feel down today, and I believe it's since things have not been going my means so possibly I need to alter something however what can I alter."

Release unfavorable emotions like temper, sadness, and also envy.

Every person manages setbacks and also disputes, and even occasionally, it's challenging to resolve the intense negative feelings that these scenarios activate. Your journal is a device that you can use to process these emotions and number out your next steps. Draw up a tirade or issue about every little thing that's going wrong. Compose a letter to the individual who hurt you yet don't send it.

Create something like, "I cannot think Alex did not give me the help she guaranteed.

I assumed I might depend on her. I wanted to chew out her until my face transforms blue. However, I do not want a bunch of drama from my mother."

Suggestion: Writing down how you feel can aid you to calm down as well as locate words you need to communicate your feelings to others. After you reveal yourself in your journal, examine what you've written and also determine what you require to do besides attend to the problem.

Track your moods every day to help you recognize your triggers.

Recording your mood in your journal entries aids you in acknowledging patterns that might lead you to your triggers. Document just how you felt throughout the day, either before or after your journal access. Additionally, rate your mood on a numerical scale. Look back over your state of mind to see what assists you feel terrific and what causes a low state of mind. This can aid you in making favorable changes to improve your mood in total.

You might write your state of mind in a word or make use of a symbol. Possible moods may consist of "satisfied," "depressing," "stressed out," "uncaring," or "mad." You could rate your moods on a scale of 1-5, with one being light as well as five being extreme. Create something like "Depressed."

Assess your entrances to help you much better comprehend your feelings.

To obtain the most out of your journaling behavior, return, and also re-read what you've created at a later time. Think about what you claimed and just how you must have been feeling. Use this to assist you in making better choices for yourself in the future. Additionally, it might aid you to reframe your thoughts so you can think in different ways regarding things in the future.

If you're undergoing a crisis, you might re-read your entry right after you wrote it or later that same day.

If you intend to enhance your general mental wellness, evaluate your posts after 3-4 months.

Using Your Journal for Self-Improvement.

Track your progression towards objectives, excellent habits, as well as positive behaviors. Use your journal to establish individual goals and also work toward favorable habits or behaviors you want to integrate into your life. Record the actions you're taking toward your objectives and check your development. Besides, make a note of or mark off when you engage in your good practices or habits.

You might maintain a page in your journal to track your development on your goal. Compose an action plan, document when you work on the objective, and check off each action.

If your goal was to meditate daily, you might block off time to practice meditation in your timetable as well as download a meditation application. After that, keep track of how frequently you meditate, the length of time your sessions last, and also the benefits you feel after reflection.

Offer yourself a sticker label or checkmark on days you work towards your goal or brand-new habits. As an example, provide yourself a face sticker label each time you do self-care, a checkmark for each glass of water you consume, or a star each day you prepare a dish in your home.

File your symptoms if you're dealing with a mental disease.

Tracking your signs and symptoms can help you identify if you're making progress or which treatments work best for you. Write down the signs you're experiencing at the top or base of your journal entrance for that day. Rate the extent of your symptoms on a mathematical range so you can better recognize them. Compare the symptoms you're experiencing with what was happening in your life that day to help you seek patterns.

You might create, "Today, I feel anxious," as well as uncertain with the numbers representing the seriousness of your symptoms.

If you're on medication, keep an eye on when you take it to see if that has any influence on your signs.

Tape proof for or versus your ideas concerning yourself.

You likely have a mix of favorable as well as adverse beliefs about yourself. Sometimes, a lot of unfavorable ideas can include in your clinical depression and stress and anxiety, even though they may not be accurate. When you have a negative thought regarding yourself, document the proof you have to both think and also disbelieve that thought.

Use this technique to help you view yourself in a more favorable light.

Let's state you think that you're foolish. You could detail examples of times you've claimed something bright, topics that you're specifically knowledgeable about, and also any education that you've completed. From there, you may state, "I'm wise when it comes to background and aiding people to organize their things."

Make a benefits and drawbacks list if you have a big decision to make.

Vast choices are always hard; however, in some cases, they can feel a lot more overwhelming if you're taking care of mental illness. Your journal can aid you to figure out what to do. Draw the line down the middle of your page, then list the pros of choice on the left side and the disadvantages on the righthand. Develop a checklist for each option you're thinking about, then choose the options that profit you the most.

You may require to make one benefits and drawbacks checklist to assist you in choosing.

For instance, let's state you're determining whether or not to obtain an emotional support animal. Pros might consist of, "Having convenience," "Never feeling alone," and "Feeling satisfied when I see my buddy." Cons could consist of "Need to clean up after it," and "Have to do paperwork."

It's practical to make multiple listings if you have several various choices. As an example, you may create numerous lists if you're determining which treatment choice to attempt.

How To Keep A Parenting Journal

Many people maintain parenting journals either to keep records for safekeeping situations or to preserve memories for their family members. While protection journals should be objective documents, journals for families need to capture the emotions related to memories. When maintaining either type of journal, however, you will wish to compose as usually as feasible and also document as much as you can.

Compose Consistently.

When keeping a parenting journal, you must write in it regularly to make it as trusted as well as authoritative as feasible. By recording information each day – or perhaps several times a day – you can be sure that what you are creating is as accurate as well as beneficial as possible.

If you write much less commonly, you run the risk of being unclear and nonspecific. You may likewise fail to remember information you meant to record.

Be Objective

While guardianship circumstances can be difficult, you require to remain as objective as possible in your parenting journal. This is not an opportunity to vent your frustrations or demonize the many other parents. Journal entrances that are certainly psychological will be less useful in a legal setting.

If you feel like you need to overcome your emotions by writing them down, attempt maintaining a separate journal or diary, that way you can express yourself without jeopardizing your custody journal.

An instance of suitable objective writing is: "John picked up our child at 4:00. The scheduled pick-up time was 3:00." An unacceptable account of the same event would state something like: "John was late once more today, like normal. He is so reckless and also a bad parent."

Keep a thorough document of your child's routine.

Your attorney will certainly require as many facts concerning your child's life and wellness as possible. To aid your attorney, keep a detailed log of what your child does daily. You can keep in mind things like medical visits, extracurricular activities, time spent with friends, and so forth — the more info you can provide the far better.

Note your role in your child's life.

Videotape when you drive them to appointments, make them meals, assist with research, and anything else you do to enhance them. You will want to ensure that your custody journal shows the crucial duty you play in your child's life.

Keep notes on all communication with the other moms and dad.

You must make a note of each time you interact with the various other parents, whether in person or online. Make a note of details regarding the moment, day, approach, as well as the length of the communication. You must additionally note the topic of the discussion, but you do not have to do so in fantastic detail.

Include of screenshots or printouts of the communication, if possible.

Track the various other parent's obligations.

You will undoubtedly wish to maintain detailed notes regarding exactly how well the various other moms and dad fulfill their obligations. Make a note of pick-up times and drop-off times. If the other moms and dad start to shirk responsibilities, take down each instance. Remember to stay objective, though.

To see to it, you continue to be objective; you ought to also keep in mind each time the other moms and dad meet responsibilities. For example, you can document something like: "Sarah took our child to the dentist today as well as brought her back home on time."

Videotape what your child states about the other parent.

Exactly how your child feels concerning the other moms and dad is extremely important, so you need to attempt to record that in addition to you can. Among the most effective methods to do this is to keep notes concerning the essential things your child claims about the other parent, using straight quotes. You do not need to require your child to say features of the other parent, yet write it down whenever the subject shows up.As always, tape the excellent along with the bad to see to it you're staying goal.

Concentrate on the child's behavior as opposed to your very own impacts. As opposed to claiming, "John is emotional as well as sad today," create, "John frowned all morning. He cried for 15 mins at 1 pm."

Track your child's mood and also habits.

To track exactly how your guardianship scenario is affecting a child's emotional health and wellness, you ought to take comprehensive notes concerning exactly how they are behaving. If a child acts in different ways than usual after being around the various other moms and dads, you can take down that.

By keeping track of your child's mental health in this way, you can also make sure that you create a custody arrangement that is ideal for them.

Videotape your child's performance in school.

You can likewise monitor your child's well-being by tape-recording their performance in school as well as any extracurricular activities. You wish to be able to determine if your custodianship plan is impacting your child's capability to succeed in school whatsoever. You need to keep in mind test ratings and progress reports, whether they are excellent or bad.If your child is having behavioral problems in school, track these as well.

Maintaining a Journal for Family Memories

Choose a writing technique you like.

You can choose to write your parenting journal in whatever way you would certainly such as. You can write with a pen or book a physical journal or create digitally on your laptop computer or tablet. One of the most important things is to select an approach that will enable you to write as frequently and also conveniently as possible. Just like a custody journal, you need to write as frequently as you can. It ensures that you can be as particular as well as detailed as possible.

Begin journaling when you know you are expecting.

If you're creating because you want to record your child's life and also share your parenting journey with your family members, you must begin as quickly as you can. The day you figure out you're expecting can be an excellent time to start a parenting journal. In this manner, you will have the ability to tape as a number of your thoughts and experiences as possible.

Track milestones.

A parenting journal is a beautiful location to tape landmarks in your child's life, such as when they take their first step or claim their very first word. Whenever anything that appears considerable happens to your child, keep in mind the occasion as well as when it occurred in your parenting journal.

You can determine what counts as a milestone however, you desire. Even if something seems relatively little, you ought to videotape it if it's essential to you as well as your child.

You can likewise use a child publication instead of an empty journal. Child books are mostly empty yet are gotten into sections devoted to developmental milestones, such as losing teeth.

Include images of significant moments in a child's life to assist in maintaining the memories even much better.

Express your feelings.

Do not merely videotape what took place during the day; define precisely how you feel concerning it. You will undoubtedly want your parenting journal to protect not just facts; also, the emotional experiences of your family members. When you blog about something charming your child has done, describe just how it made you feel. It will undoubtedly make your journal a touching record a period in your family's life that passes promptly.

Someday, your children will read this journal and will undoubtedly wonder to learn about what you were like currently. The even more details regarding your mood you can give, the extra you can satisfy that inquisitiveness.

Focus on the favorable.

You don't require to stay away from unfavorable topics entirely, yet you do not wish to dwell on them. Being as well negative could injure the sensations of your child if you wind up sharing the journal with them. You intend to make sure you're focusing mainly on the happy moments that you as well as your child, share.

Show your journal to your child when they're ready.

Among the objectives of a family, parenting journal is to be able to utilize it to reveal your children what their very early life was like, as they will have no memories of it. Whenever you feel your child prepares to see what you've created and recorded, you can share it with them.

If you've written a great deal concerning yourself as well as your emotions, you may want to wait until your child is older.

SIMPLE HINTS AND POINTERS FOR AVOIDING MELTDOWN

1. Pinpoint the source.

Psychotherapist Stephanie Sarkis, Ph.D., recommended looking "at what might be causing your child's actions." When you can locate the source of the habits, she said, you can make strides towards changing it.

Knowing what triggers your child, Matlen stated, can assist you in defusing their tantrum as very early as possible. For instance, is your child starving? Are they sleep-deprived? Are they experiencing stable emotions? As soon as you pinpoint the underlying problem, attempt to solve it, she stated.

Additionally, it is an excellent device for protecting against temper tantrums. If your child cannot manage the overstimulating environment of a neighborhood fair, don't take them, as stated by Matlen.

2. Explain the consequences in advance.

Before a temper tantrum ever starts, Matlen recommended talking with your child regarding the unfavorable consequences of negative behaviors. She provided this instance: "If you yell as well as weep when I switch off the TV, you won't be able to enjoy it later today."

Matlen took this strategy when her little girl was five years old. She tended to have temper tantrums when she did not get a brand-new toy at the shop. "Before our next outing, I informed her that if she had an outburst, I would pick her up and take her home. No toys and also no more trips to the store for a very long time."

Her daughter still had a meltdown. However, as opposed to getting angry or frustrated, Matlen picked up her child as well as took her to the vehicle. She drove home without stating a word as well as it never occurred once more.

" This, of course, might not work for all children, yet it's an example of intending in advance and also having an outcome that every person comprehends."

3. Talk with your child, as well as urge them to discuss.

Talk smoothly as well as quietly to your child, and recognize their feelings, Matlen stated. Doing so helps your child feel listened to, Sarkis claimed.

According to Matlen, you could state, "I recognize you're angry that I won't buy you that toy today. It feels frustrating, and it makes you seem like taking off inside, does not it?"

Then, urge your child to express their feelings, also: "I 'd be distressed also if I could not obtain what I wanted right now – let's talk about why this is so vital to you so you can help me to understand."

4. Sidetrack your child.

For younger children, distraction might work, Matlen stated. "Talk concerning something completely different, like exactly how thrilled you are to enjoy the TV program you intended when you all get home."

5. Give them a break.

" Sometimes, absolutely nothing seems to work, though, and also a child will certainly not quit regardless of what you attempt," Matlen said. When that occurs, comfortably clarify that they'll need to visit their area. They can appear after they've calmed down. It is an effective way to learn self-soothing actions, she stated. As a result of that, it's crucial to maintain items that advertise healthy copings, such as a teddy bear or fidget toys, she added.

6. Overlook the tantrum.

"Sometimes the very best response to an outburst is no response," said Sarkis, writer of numerous publications on ADHD, consisting of *"Making the Grade with ADD: A Student's Guide to Succeeding in School with Attention Deficit Disorder."* That's because "even unfavorable interest is the focus, as well as it provides a 'reward' for the actions." So not offering your child a "target market" could assist in decreasing the size of the outburst.

If your child has an outburst in the center of the shop – and it's not crowded – let them have the tantrum, Sarkis said. "You might get looks from others. It's ALRIGHT. Just bear in mind that not paying attention to the habits assists to extinguish it."

7. Provide tips.

According to both experts, children with ADHD have a hard time with shifts. They can have a meltdown when it's time to leave the play area or stop playing their videogame to have dinner, Matlen claimed. "Things that are enjoyable are hard to quit, especially when the transition is into a task they might not appreciate."

This is when pointers are essential. For example, remind your child at 30, 15, 10, and five-minute intervals that supper is ready, Matlen claimed. Additionally, establish appropriate consequences if they do not conform, such as not playing videogames after dinner, or playing them for 15 minutes as opposed to 30, she stated (or just restriction videogames before dinner entirely).

Matlen provided this instance of what to claim to your child: "I recognize it's difficult for you to stop playing your PlayStation when it's time for supper. I will provide you reminders so that you can wind down. Nevertheless, having a temper tantrum is not acceptable, so if that happens, you will certainly (fill in the space)."

8. Commend your child when they do show self-control.

"Parents require to catch their children being great far more than they capture them being 'bad,'" Sarkis stated. "Children with ADHD react well to positive support." Also, "whatever you focus on grows," she added.

According to Matlen, rather than saying, "You are such an excellent young boy for not having a meltdown when I said no to ice cream," a much better response would undoubtedly be, "You have to have truly felt pleased with yourself that you did not have a tantrum when you saw that we were out of cookies – excellent job!"

9. Avoid corporal penalties.

It's a typical response to snap when a moms and dad sees his/her child flat out on the flooring lashing out, kicking as well as screaming," Matlen said. You might grab your child or perhaps spank them. However, this only gas the negative situation as well as every person's feelings, she claimed. "Corporal penalty might soothe the behavior temporarily –though normally, it just raises the negative behavior – yet it additionally establishes the tone that it's OKAY to hit people when you're mad." Also, a child requires to "get himself in control."

Taking care of tantrums is difficult. By planning, staying calm as well as applying particular methods, you can appease them. Also, if the temper tantrum does not go silent, try to ride it out.

Precisely How To Prevent After-School Meltdowns

As moms and dad, you may observe that your child leaves for school packed with joy and also gets back under a dark cloud. They may blast you, toss a tantrum, or have a full meltdown after school. It is called "after-school restraint collapse," and it occurs because the school can be mentally draining. Therefore, they may be in a weary, irritated state of mind when they get to the house. You can prevent after-school crises by producing a regular for your child to adhere to and also by maintaining them calm as quickly as they enter the door. If your child has an after-school meltdown, you need steps to moderate the situation as well as ease them.

Identify that troubles during school can cause bottled-up anxiety.

School can be a challenging experience for some children. Handling their emotions and impulses is hard work.

They might keep their feelings shut in until they reach a place where they feel secure. (The excellent news is that your child does feel safe in your home, or they would not discharge their emotions).

Understand variables that make some children extra susceptible to meltdowns after school.

Age, perfectionism, and also impairments can cause children having a more difficult time dealing with the stress and anxiety of school.

Age plays a role in after-school disasters. Younger children are less mentally resilient and, therefore, more likely to have a meltdown. They are expected to grow out of these disasters.

Perfectionism can make a child seem like they need to be "best" at school.Therefore, they may be an angel at school, only to break down in pieces once they get home.

Impairments like dyslexia or autism can suggest that children require added assistance at school, as well as they might not always get sufficient aid. They may also be rejected or criticized unfairly by peers or teachers.

Recognize that severe or regular after-school disasters might signify a much deeper issue.

If your child's meltdowns are unusually horrible or frequent, after that, it may suggest that things aren't okay at school. Your child might be handling an issue like:

- Bullying.
- A mean instructor.
- Frustrating schoolwork.
- Too much stress to perform.
- Stress and anxiety issues.
- Lack of ample assistance for special needs (diagnosed or undiagnosed).

Speak up if you believe that something is seriously incorrect.

If your child's disasters look like they are abnormally regular or extreme, then that indicates that there can be an underlying issue. Do not wait it out. Instead, ask other people concerning what's going on.

Ask your child: what makes school hard? What is the hardest component of school? What are theother children like?

Ask other moms and dads: do their children have similar disasters, or make your child's meltdowns sound even worse than average?

Ask your child's teachers: what takes place at school that could be creating so much anxiety? Exist in any social or academic troubles? Does your child seem to be having a problem with stress and anxiety administration?

Ask your child's pediatrician: are these crises normal for their age, or could the child be experiencing an emotional handicap?

Creating an After-School Routine.

Welcome your child with a smile, as well as no questions.

When your child gets home from school, avoid annoying them with great deals of questions about their day or just how they feel. Conserve the concerns for a later time when they are resolved and also relaxed. Instead, greet them with a smile as well as a "welcome home" or a "great to have you back." Be cozy and also positive when they walk through the door, so they begin to feel much more loosened up as well as tranquil.

You can also try asking your child, "Do you intend to discuss your day now or later on?" They have the alternative to informing you about their day currently or at a later time. This will show them that you appreciate their day yet comprehend they may be bewildered and also require a long time to unwind before you speak.

Have treats or a meal ready for them.

Many children get back from schools hungry, as well as hunger integrated with irritability or fatigue can cause a tiff. Avoid a meltdown by providing them treats or a tiny dish right when they get home. You can likewise put some snacks out in a bowl in the kitchen area so they can access them on their own.

If the drive from the school to your home is a long one, bring a snack so your child can consume it on the playground or in the vehicle on the way home.

You may prepare healthy treats like cut-up fruit or a dish of nuts. You can also leave out crackers or chips for your child to snack on when they get home from school, so they please their appetite yet not spoil their appetite for supper.

Let your child have some downtime alone.

You should additionally make downtime part of your child's after-school regimen, where they can take a break as well as have time to themselves. Giving your child an hour of downtime once they get to the house can aid them to relax and also release several of the anxiousness or tension of their school day.

You may offer your child an hour to themselves in their room where they can use their computer, listen to music, or review.

Your child may likewise favor being active as a component of their downtime where they play a sporting activity outside or run about in the yard for an hour after school.

If your child appears exhausted, supply a chance for them to take a nap.

Prepare your child for homework or dinner.

As a component of your child's after-school routine, you need to additionally prepare your child for homework at night as well as dinnertime. Provide a half an hour to an hour to themselves, and after that, remind them that they must start their homework in the next 15 minutes to an hour. You also need to allow them to recognize what time dinner will be so they can plan for it. In this manner, they feel much less worried as well as can stay with a regular routine.

As an example, you may inform your child, "How regarding we do research in 30 mins together at the cooking area table?" or "Remember that dinner is in an hour, fine?".

Keeping Your Child Calm After School.

Establish a calm atmosphere for them.

An additional way you can prevent your child from having a meltdown when they get home from school is to create a residence atmosphere that is tranquil as well as kicking back for them. Prevent having great deals of mess everywhere in your house and also keep the noise degree down. Clean the common area and also lay out your child's plaything, so they are simple to access when they get home from school.

You might also attempt to establish a tranquil setting for yourself as well, such as lighting candle lights, placing on relaxing music, and even doing a relaxing task before your child gets home. It could, after that, help you to set a calm tone for your child when they walk through the door.

Do enjoyable, involving activities with your child.

You can likewise keep your child's spirits up when they get to the house by providing to do some fun activities with them when they get home. Possibly you set up a craft location where you can draw and also paint with each other. Or perhaps, you bring out your child's favored parlor game and also recommend you play around together. It can help your child remain involved and also work off any adverse energy they are bringing home with them.

You may say to your child, "How concerning we get imaginative and do some crafts before homework?" or "Do you intend to play a board game before dinner?"

Enable them to play with brothers or sisters or friends.

You ought to additionally urge your child to burn off any negative power from school by playing with brothers or sisters or friends. Possibly your child has a neighborhood good friend nearby that they like to run around with outside. Or probably your child invites a close friend over to hang around in their space after school. Let them have good friends over so they can destress and also have fun.

For example, you may state to your child, "Do you want to invite a buddy over to play?" or "Would you such as to go have fun with your friend across the street?".

Recognize your child's sensations.

If your child does have an after-school meltdown, you must be prepared for it and also handle it as necessary. Start by recognizing your child's feelings. They are likely feeling tired, stressed out, as well as irritated. Comfort them that you understand they are exhausted from school and lashing out because they are worried. Doing this can aid to deescalate the situation and also allow them to recognize you are on their side.

For instance, you may state to your child, "We're tired out from school, aren't we?" or "You had a long day, didn't you? You're all set to have a snack and also relax."

A visual sensations graph would undoubtedly be useful if your child is still discovering how to connect their feelings.

Separate your child from others.

If there are various other children in your home, you should have your child transfer to a separate location, such as their bedroom. It will give them an area to cool down and also take a couple of deep breaths. Have them stay in their space for five to ten minutes, as this will certainly provide a chance to cool down as well as be on their very own.

Often, some alone time in a safe room like their room can assist them to unwind and release any tension from school.

It is likewise an excellent way to stay clear of distressing the other children and help to maintain a calm area for everyone else in your household.

Offer your child time and also the area to relax by themselves.

Instead of trying to fix your child's issue for them or snap at them, let them calm down on their own. You might leave them with their toys or books as well as a tiny treat. After a few minutes, they must calm down and come to be engaged in a plaything or their snack.

As soon as your child has cooled down as well as the meltdown has passed, you may then inquire concerning their day at school or ask if they 'd like to have fun with you. Involve with them just after they have relaxed.

DECREASING YOUR STRESS DEGREES ON ADHD – IS IT POSSIBLE?

If you have ADHD, you might have difficulty with socializing, listening abilities, as well as focusing. It can result in a lot of stress as well as frustration. It's all-natural to have a tough time when every day could seem like a fight.

Right here are some ways to manage your stress.

Practice deep breathing.

This strategy loads a one-two punch by reducing ADHD signs as well as reducing stress and anxiety. Discovering to use your breath to your advantage can aid you to boost leisure and also boost attention. Deep breathing jumpstarts your body's all-natural stress feedback, assisting you to end up being more secure.

Situate a place where you can be in peace for several minutes without disturbance. Sit down comfortably and also close your eyes. Breathe in genuinely and also gradually via your nose, ensuring that your stomach is expanding with each inhales. Release the air by exhaling through your mouth, noticing your stubborn belly deflating like a balloon. Repeat this exercise numerous times

Discover mindfulness.

It may appear not likely for a person with ADHD to successfully practice mindfulness. Still, the study shows it is really possible as well as likewise effective at decreasing signs and symptoms. Mindfulness is the practice of concentrating on the present moment, which can be a significant obstacle for individuals with ADHD. Researches show that mindfulness training can help improve focus. What's even more, mindfulness techniques are also efficient at minimizing stress and tension and anxiety.

To practice mindfulness, find a quiet location where you can sit comfortably for around 15 to 20 minutes without disturbances. Unwind your arm or legs. Shut your eyes and take a breath generally. Currently, start deep breathing, taking long, sluggish inhales in with your nose. Then, exhale slowly through your mouth. You can count emotionally as well as state "One." Repeat. Whenever you discover that your ideas have strayed, return your focus to your breath as well as restart your being at one again.

Understanding mindfulness to get rid of ADHD yourself can be quite severe. Speak with your psychotherapist or mental wellness provider regarding completing a mindfulness training program under specialist supervision.

Relieve tension in your body.

If you are feeling stressed out, there are likely indications of stress in your body. Progressive muscular tissue relaxation instructs you exactly how to utilize your organization to lower pressure. This exercise can be included in a deep breathing practice for dual the advantage.

Do this workout in a quiet, secluded area. Lie down pleasantly on a couch or a bed. Relax your muscle mass as well as take several deep, cleansing breaths. Gradually relocate through each significant muscle group in your body, having and then releasing the muscle mass.

Begin at your temple.

Scrunch up your forehead as well as curve your eyebrows for a couple of seconds. Release the stress and also discover how it feels when the pressure goes away. Transfer to the next muscular tissue team until you have completed your entire body. Once the exercise is completed, you should feel both emotionally and also literally relaxed.

Set up in time for play or relaxation.

Not having special times to look after yourself or locate satisfaction establishes you up for exhaustion at school or work. Make time weekly (or each day, if possible) to engage in a task that you locate pleasurably. It may consist of strolling on the beach, having fun with your pet dog, watching a preferred funny motion picture, or baking cookies. Make time to do what you like typically.

Be patient with yourself. Don't beat yourself up.

Recognize that you are dealing with a severe mental condition in which you will undoubtedly make mistakes. If you hold yourself to the criterion of people without ADHD, you will always feel like a failure.

Instead, offer yourself a break and celebrate the small successes that you accomplish in a day. These may consist of getting to a function or school promptly or remembering to jot down your research or tasks listing.

Advocate yourself.

Being conscious of your needs as well as using your voice can help you lessen excess stress in the long haul. Successfully fighting ADHD and stress and anxiety call for that you end up being experienced about both problems and your constraints. When you know yourself as well as your demands, you are much better geared up to communicate those needs to others.

Educate yourself extensively regarding both ADHD and also stress and anxiety as well as know the signs and symptoms of each. Speak up at school or the workplace if you are being asked to carry out in a way that is tough for you as a result of these problems.

As an example, if you have trouble taking examinations within an arranged time, you may need to consult with your school concerning getting test-taking accommodations. Raise your hand or draw your teacher aside and state, "Ms. Winters, it's stressful for me to complete my test in 45 minutes. Can you work with me to ensure that I do not feel so much anxiousness about taking examinations?"

Discover to identify and also stay clear of triggers.

You automatically really feel a lot more efficient in managing stress and anxiousness related to ADHD when you can acknowledge what's creating it. Fears, clutter, as well as still time are all potential triggers.

When you have determined your triggers, take a seat, and come up with options to ensure that you can prevent them entirely. If idle time appears to set off anxiousness in you, it can be valuable to develop an everyday timetable that maintains you valid and active while consisting of a list of recreation activities you can do throughout your free time. In this way, you won't need to feel stressed out concerning downtime; you can merely take part in one of your set tasks throughout that time.

Get systems in position to counteract organizational concerns.

You may be against developing a routine but doing so can aid profoundly. Produce a feeling of structure in your life that aids you reduce stress and also decreases lack of organization.

As an example, you could invest some time each night getting prepared for the following with day

Lay out your clothes. Collect any essential files, such as types or projects.

You can likewise create a system for arranging documentation that has remained as well as finishing homework. Talk to your school psychotherapist, psychological health and wellness service providers, or educators to see if they can suggest any valuable systems for you to implement into daily life.

Manage your time efficiently.

A person with ADHD may have trouble assessing time and handling target dates. If you recognize that this is an obstacle for you, research methods to use to boost your time-management abilities.

These may consist of establishing timers that tell you when to quit one task as well as the move to an additional. Or, you may require to develop suggestions on your phone so that you do not forget crucial consultations or events. Recognize your restrictions as well as place steps in the position that aid you.

Take breaks when needed.

Stress can be developing as well as you did not also notice it. To effectively take care of anxiety, you need to have all-natural breaks into your day that enable you to see the tension and alleviate it before it takes place.

Every hour approximately, time out as well as take inventory of how your body feels. Is stress present? Is your heart racing? Are you feeling overwhelmed? Are your ideas negative?

If you spot the signs of mounting stress, act, close your eyes, and take several full minutes of deep breathing. Stretch your legs and go for a walk in nature. Call a buddy for a fast conversation. It's essential to discover when you're feeling stressed out as well as implement procedures to decrease it as necessary.

Following up with Treatment

Speak with your medical professional about using stimulants appropriately.

Although stimulant medications have shown to be highly effective in dealing with the signs of ADHD, this benefit does not come without expense. Stimulants have the power to trigger or get worse existing stress and anxiety signs and symptoms.

Some medical professionals state that the stress and anxiety felt while taking stimulants takes place as the body adjusts to the medication, which symptoms should decrease in the coming days and weeks. All the same, your doctor can also recommend a non-stimulant in conjunction with a Selective Serotonin Reuptake Inhibitor(SSRI) for people who cannot tolerate stimulant drugs.

Another option is to take a drug to treat among the disorder (i.e., the ADHD or the anxiousness) and manage the various other with behavioral and lifestyle changes.

Attempt treatment if it helps.

Trying to deal with either ADHD or anxiousness with drugs only may not demonstrate optimal outcomes. Individuals must think about global lifestyle modifications in enhancement to various other specialist therapies, such as action therapy.

Behavior therapy is a treatment strategy helped with by a doctor, school psychotherapist, or various other psychological health and wellness providers to improve the more subtle signs and symptoms of ADHD. A structured program is developed that makes use of incentives and also consequences to boost abilities and remove unwanted behavior patterns.

Adjusting your diet plan as necessary.

There is no clear evidence that diet and also dietary shortages create ADHD or anxiousness; there is evidence to show positive modifications can boost signs in both disorders. Foods that help the mind are helpful for individuals with ADHD.

These include a wealth of proteins discovered in meat, poultry, beans, nuts, as well as cheese. Eat much less simple carbohydrates like sugar, white flour, and white rice as well as even more complicated carbohydrates located in fruits, vegetables, and also whole grains. Foods with omega-3 fatty acids likewise help, such as salmon and also walnuts.

Nutritional supplements may likewise lower signs. Consider taking a 100% minerals and vitamin supplement daily.

Exercise frequently.

You might currently have received a suggestion to apply a regimen of exercise from your primary care medical professional. Regular exercise helps develop strong bones and also muscle mass. Nevertheless, along with physical fitness, exercise additionally assists the mind.

Neurotransmitters, select chemicals in mind, are created during exercise that can decrease inattention and also enhance cognitive reasoning abilities. An included advantage is that exercise also reduces stress and even anxiety.

The majority of doctors recommend a minimum of 30 minutes of moderate-intensity workout on many of days in a week.

HOW REGULAR EXERCISE CAN HELP YOUR CHILD'S BEHAVIOR

You might have currently heard that regular exercise can give your state of mind an increase. If you have ADHD, an exercise does more than make you feel great. It can help regulate your symptoms, also.

Even a single session of moving your body can make you more inspired for mental tasks, raise your psychic ability, give you energy, and also help you feel less confused. It acts upon your brain in a lot of similarities as your ADHD medication.

To reap these benefits, however, you are required to exercise the proper way as well as the correct amount. The trick is to discover an activity that fits your lifestyle and then persevere.

Get the Most out of Moving Around

The results of exercise last for so long, much like medicine. Consider your workout as a therapy "dose." Go for at the very least one 30- to 40-minute task a day, four or five days a week.

The exercise you choose depends on you, but make sure it's "reasonably extreme," which means that during your workout:

- Your heart rate rises
- You take a breath more challenging and also quicker
- You sweat
- Your muscular tissues feel exhausted

Talk to your doctor if you're unclear how intense your exercise should be. She may recommend you utilize a heart rate screen or some other tool to make sure you obtain one of the most out of your workout.

Types of Exercise You Can Do

Aerobic exercise. It is anything that gets your heart pounding. You wish to do something that elevates your heart rate and also maintains it there for a set quantity of time, like half an hour to 40 minutes.

Cardiovascular exercise develops new pathways in your mind as well as floods it with the chemicals that help you listen.

You can attempt among these:

- Running

- Strolling quickly
- Cycling
- Swimming laps

You can do these tasks outdoors or inside, but if you have an option, go outside. Researches show that remaining in nature while you move can reduce your ADHD signs and symptoms a lot more than when you exercise within.

Martial arts. Experts say the extra complex your exercise is, the far better for your mind. Sports like martial arts, taekwondo, jiujitsu, as well as judo focus on self-discipline as well as bringing together your mind and body. When you do martial arts, you obtain training in abilities like:

- Focus and attention
- Equilibrium
- Timing
- Memory
- Effects of activities
- Fine motor abilities

Other complex exercises. If fighting styles aren't your thing, other physical activities that also challenge your mind and body are:

- Rock climbing
- Dance

- Gymnastics
- Yoga

Strength training. If you're only just starting with exercise, go for cardio activities like strolling or jogging. After you've gone to it for some time, add in some stamina work for range. Attempt workouts like:

- Lunges
- Squats
- Pushups
- Pullups
- Weight training

Team sporting activities. If you join a softball or football organization, it may be merely the thing to get you up and also moving several times a week. Organized sports have all the benefits of exercise with the added benefit of a social team to motivate you.

Team effort refines your communication skills as well as aids you in analyzing your activities and also strategy in advance. Being part of a group can additionally enhance your self-worth.

How to Keep at It

Much like medication, exercise helps you treat ADHD if you keep it up. If you have issues with the focus span, how do you remain the course?

Try these ideas:

1. Keep it interesting. Switch over the type of exercise. You can stay out of a rut if you alter your activity daily or weekly.
2. Locate a partner. An exercise buddy can help you stay on track as well as help kill time while you sweat.
3. Move-in the morning. If it fits in your routine, exercise first thing in the early morning before you take your medication. That way, you'll get the most gain from all the extra mood-boosting chemicals in your body.
4. Maintain meds. Exercise can give you a substantial upper hand on your ADHD signs. However, it does not change your medication. Do not stop your other therapies unless your doctor claims it's alright.

How To Help Children Manage ADHD With Yoga

Attention Deficit Disorder (ADHD) is a condition that appears in early childhood, with signs and symptoms that generally appear before the age of seven.

If your child has ADHD or you collaborate with children with ADHD, you might take into consideration trying different therapies like yoga. Yoga has been shown in research studies to be an appealing treatment for children with ADHD.

You can do yoga exercises at home with children with ADHD or obtain a professional yoga instructor. You should, after that, create a yoga exercise routine so the child can reap the benefits of this technique.

Educate your child to identify sensations in their body. Various feelings and also degrees of power will be felt differently by your child. They may feel like they have butterflies in their belly or are buzzing with electricity at times when they're hyper. Conversely, they may feel lighter sometimes when they're loosened up. Discovering to see these sensations will help them see exactly how yoga exercise affects them.

Ask your child to rank their energy degree on a scale of 1 to 10 before and after yoga. It will undoubtedly help them see the advantages.

Make yoga enjoyable for your child.

Attach the yoga to something that your child delights in to ensure that they'll be much more open up to trying it. For instance, you might call it "superhero training" to interest a child that likes superheroes. You might even relabel the positions to make them sound more enjoyable to your child.

Teach your children to enjoy their breath.

Being aware of their breath will undoubtedly help your child experience the full benefits of yoga. Initially, instruct your child to monitor their breathing. Once they get used to that, you can guide them just how to breathe in and exhale with each move.

Show them how to extend their breath by gradually inhaling.

Describe just how they can strengthen their breaths by pulling the air right into their tummy as well as lungs. Inform them that it takes technique, so they should do their best.

Concentrate on movement-based yoga.

After you show your child to check their breath, show them just how to relocate via the poses. Ask your child to imitate an animal, transferring through poses like cat pose, downward dog, roaring lion position, and cobra pose. Urge them to relocate slow activity, watching their breath.

Doing Yoga In Your Home

Begin with the Mountain Pose.

Mountain pose is a great introductory move that you can do with children with ADHD. Place a yoga mat in an open space in your home and also start the yoga session with Mountain pose to help the child concentrate on the practice.

To show the child exactly how to do Mountain Pose, stand straight with your feet close to each other. Open and also spread your toes, so they are level on the mat. Straighten your legs without locking at the knees.

Bend down by pressing through your big toes and also raise your head, keeping your face forward and even your head level. Place your hands by your sides with your hands available to the front of the room.

Hold the Mountain position for ten deep inhales and breathes out. You might have the childcount the breaths with you to keep them focused.

Practice the Roaring Lion Pose.

Roaring Lion position is a simple yoga exercise pose that can help your child relax and also have a good time on the mat. The concept is to roar like a lion in the jungle in this pose, making the most vicious face you can summon.

To do this posture with the child, kneel on the yoga exercise mat with your bottom hand on your calves. Position your hands on your knees and stay upright.

Open your mouth as well as close your eyes. Extend your tongue out as well as down, wrinkling your nose. Inhale and afterward, as you breathe out, release a "ROARRRR" sound.

Repeat this sound five times for five breaths in total. It can be fun to do this position before a mirror, as you shout at your very own image.

Do the Tree Pose.

Tree pose benefits focus and concentration. It is likewise an excellent challenge for children with ADHD to stay concentrated enough to maintain their balance.

Begin by standing with your palms along with your thumbs at your breastbone. Keep your hands together and also slowly increase your hands over your head. Lower them back down to the beginning placement. Repeat this several times, integrating your breathing with an upward movement and also your respiration with a descending motion.

Add on the harmonizing element by focusing on an unmoving spot on the floor four feet far from you. Extend your right leg and also place your right foot against your left calf, with your bent leg facing the right side.

Hold this pose for five breaths and afterward release. Switch over to the other side, lifting your left foot as well as placing it against your right calf.

Practice the Superman Pose.

This posture can help the child come to be a lot more aware of their body language as well as feel more grounded. They might also enjoy the experience of "flying" on the ground.

To do Superman Pose, relax on your belly with your arms stretched overhead and your legs straight behind you. Start by inhaling as well as raising your arms off the ground. Exhale and also place your arms back on the ground. Do the very same with your legs, lifting and lowering your legs with your take a breath.

As soon as the child appears comfortable with training and also decreasing their arm or legs, you can attempt the complete posture. Inhale as well as lift both your limbs off the ground. You need to seem like you're flying like a superhero. Breathe out and also lower your arm or legs. Repeat this pose for 4 to 5 complete breaths.

Attempt the Drawbridge Pose.

This pose is good for focusing the child as well as permitting them to have even more control over the motion of their body. It is an excellent pose to likewise help your childunwind, especially if they seem to be getting flustered or active.

Begin by pushing your back with your arms at hand, and your palms down. Bend your knees and also put your feet flat on the ground. They must be hip-width apart and close enough that you can touch your heels with your hands.

Inhale as you press firmly right into your feet and also hands. Lift your hips off the ground like the raising of a drawbridge. After that, breathe out as you lower your hips down to the floor.

Repeat this pose for four to five breaths. As soon as you are done, hug your knees to your chest for five to 10 breaths.

Relax with Child's Pose.

This pose is fantastic for concluding a yoga session or as a last yoga posture before bed. You can show the child to enter into this pose if they start to feel overloaded or hyper, as it can be extremely relaxing as well as relaxing.

To do Child's Pose, stoop down and sit on your feet with your knees divided. You might allow your knees to develop a broad "v" form on the floor covering. Inhale and put your forehead on the ground before your knees, curving your back. Prolong your arms ahead and also take a breath genuinely in this pose for two to five minutes.

Begin of the pose gradually, lifting your arms and also head. Relax on your feet as well as take a few cleansing breaths to finish your practice.

Getting Professional Yoga Instruction

Seek a yoga exercise course for children with ADHD in your area.

Not all yoga exercise educators will undoubtedly be experienced sufficient to deal with children with

ADHD. You need to search for a yoga exercise class instructed by an instructor who has a strong foundation in yoga and also is familiar with how to communicate with people with ADHD. The teacher may be accredited to deal with developmentally tested children or have substantial experience mentoringchildren with ADHD.

The majority of yoga courses for children with ADHD will have two to threechildren at once. It will enable the yoga exercise educator to function patiently as well as very carefully with each child.

Watch yoga exercise videos online.

You can obtain expert yoga exercise guidelines on a budget by searching for yoga exercise videos online that focus on poses for people with ADHD. You may register for a couple of video channels on the internet so you can see brand-new video clips weekly and integrate them right into yoga exercise sessions with the child.

You may likewise ask parents or teachers who deal with children with ADHD for recommendations on yoga video channels or websites.

Hire a private yoga exercise teacher.

You may select hiring a yoga instructor for private lessons for the child, so they get one on one focus. Try to find a yoga trainer who is accredited to show children with ADHD and also who has worked with children with ADHD before. The teacher needs to appear, in person, confident, and even open with the child in the one on one sessions.

The instructor might also include quick routines in their sessions, like illumination incense or setting up a floor covering, so the child gets used to concentrating on detailed tasks. They may then do a collection of poses, making an effort to get the child to focus as well as relax during the session.

Developing a Yoga Routine

Have a deep breathing session daily.

Starting a yoga exercise routine with the child can benefit them over time. It can likewise make them comfier with doing yoga and also in time, get even more self-confidence. You may start by setting aside time in the child's schedule to do deep breathing once daily. In-depth breathing sessions can be an excellent way to help your child focus and unwind. They can, after that, make use of deep breaths when they are doing yoga poses.

You can sit with the child in a peaceful, darkened space in a comfortable position to do deep breathing. Try to do at the very least 10 to fifteen slow deep inhales as well as exhales. You might have the child place one hand on their belly and also one hand on their chest to help them get used to breathing in and breathing out deeply.

Do a couple of yoga exercises poses before bed.

You may also urge the child to do a couple of relaxing yoga poses before they go to bed. You may do them together as a component of the child's bedtime routine. Doing unwinding positions before bed can help the child settle down and also get in rest mode.

Make this enjoyable for your child! You could show them to do a couple of postures before bed to "trigger sleep mode," after that, a few poses in the morning to "trigger wake setting."

You might do Mountain Pose, Drawbridge Pose, and also Child's Pose together before bed. Make sure you synchronize your activities with your inhales and exhaling out.

Set up the standard once a week yoga session.

You need to attempt to have once a week yoga sessions with the child, so they obtain used to doing the yoga exercise positions as well as more positive doing them. You might register the child in a regular yoga exercise course for children with ADHD or schedule an exclusive yoga exercise session.

You may also have your very own sessions at home with the child, so they get used to doing yoga at the very least once a week.

Do yoga exercise outside to help the child focused.

If you discover the child is having difficulties focusing on the yoga exercise poses, you may attempt moving the session outside. Studies have shown that children with ADHD have far better focus when they are outdoors in natural, environment-friendly atmospheres.

You might move the yoga exercise sessions to your yard or an eco-friendly space by your home. You might likewise attempt to have a few of the yoga sessions inside as well as some sessions outdoors, so the child feels they have variety.

Differ, the yoga poses you make with the child.

Children with ADHD succeed with energetic, differed activities. They tend to get tired quickly and come to be distracted as soon as they have lost interest in a task. You can keep the child focused by doing various yoga postures, or the same yoga poses in a different order during the yoga exercise sessions.

You may also attempt to include other exercises with yoga, so the child feels tested and boosted.

If you take the child to a yoga exercise class, make sure the trainer differs the yoga poses performed in the class week to week, so the child remains engaged.

Encourage your child to fine tune their positions.

WHY A SIMPLE CHANGE IN ATTITUDE MAY WORK WONDERS?

As a parent, you certainly enjoy your children. However, you may become annoyed when they misbehave. Children will undoubtedly act out as a method to seek attention, press limits, or to mimic the habits of others. On top of that, children require advice creating their coping skills to handle their emotions; when that is lacking, your children might act out. Your child may act out in troublesome times or in devastating means, which can be tiring. Taking steps in the direction of changing and also enhancing your children' poor habits will be beneficial for your children in both the short as well as long-term, while likewise making your life simpler.

Connect Your Expectations For Your Child's Behavior.

Children require to understand what you expect from them. Rest your child down in a peaceful location and also clarify to him/her what sort of behaviors you intend to see, using clear information. Concentrate on correcting one habit each time. Giving your child a lengthy listing of items for improvement can be frustrating.

Tell him/her things like, "When you are at school, you need to listen to your teacher," or you could state, "I do not desire you to strike other children, also if they are mean to you."

Set Realistic Expectations

Set high assumptions for your children, but not so high they are unreachable. You want your children to have to function as well as think of what you expect. However, they must likewise be able to achieve what you are asking from them. Or else, they may seem like failings and also deal with minimized self-confidence. You also need to make sure that your assumptions are age-appropriate.

Establish an expectation like "I expect you to turn up to class promptly as well as be considerate to your teachers," rather than "I anticipate you to be a straight-A student."

Anticipating your four-year-old never to lose his/her temper is unrealistic. However, expecting him/her to control his/her temper and not hit other children is sensible.

Follow your very own rules.

Children see what you do and will undoubtedly tend to duplicate your actions as well as actions. If they see you disregarding to follow an expectation you made, they will undoubtedly presume they can ignore it.

Bear in mind that children usually discover by example. For that reason, if you shout instead of going over things with them, then they will most likely embrace these actions. Or, if you do disappoint regard for authority figures, then your children may likewise demonstrate comparable disrespect for their teachers, coaches, moms and dads of their pals, and even you.

Keep your expectations consistent for each scenario.

Remain active and do not transform the assumption for each different circumstance. Hold your children to the very same standard, whether they are going to school, church, or the supermarket. Refer back to your composed checklist of assumptions before every new occasion to guarantee both you and your child recognize what is expected.

For example, if you have set a "no outbursts" plan, do not give in if your child throws a temper tantrum in the supermarket. Follow up with whatever consequences you have set. If you change your assumption to get your child to stop the negative actions, he/she will undoubtedly discover that he/she can push your limitations by misbehaving.

Consistency constructs trust bonds between you as well as your child. It will help frame you as dependable, and also reinforce the bond between both of you.

Uniformity will also help reduce "assuming" how your child may feel regarding how to behave in specific scenarios, making them a lot more protected as well as most likely to act much better.

Do not negotiate your assumptions with your children.

You are the parent, so you have to set as well as adhere to the regulations you make. If your child negotiates with you, advise him/her that what is anticipated of him/her has been set out, as well as he/she is responsible for promoting what you have discussed.

If you have established the assumption that your child has to finish his/her homework before he/she can play his/her video game, you need not let him attempt to negotiate his/her way out of doing his/her homework.

If you provide into discussing with your children, you immediately stop corresponding. If your children realize they can negotiate with you about what is anticipated of them, they will not take you or the behavioral assumptions seriously.

Nevertheless, it's additionally essential to take notice of the scenario. If your boy is arguing regarding not cleaning his/her teeth, ask him/her why he/she doesn't desire to. You could learn that he has a loose tooth that injures when he/she brushes it. Lots of children say when they don't recognize how else to share their sensations, especially sensations of discomfort or frustration.

Maintain in mind that arrangement can be a positive thing when your children get older. It can boost communication between you and your teen as well as make it much easier to understand each other. Allowing your teenager to negotiate, you can also advertise vital thinking and even diplomacy. Also, it does not mean that you have to give up, just that you need to agree to pay attention.

Transforming Bad Behavior

Be proactive! Stopping poor actions before it also begins is essential.

Discover the patterns of your child's actions so you can be prepared to do something about it. If you recognize your child is going to call for your focus throughout an essential phone call, involve her in a challenge or a TV show that will hold her interest for the duration of your telephone call.

Be clear with your child, informing her specifically what is going to take place. Before your phone call, state something like, "Mommy will certainly be on the phone for 10 mins. I require you not to disrupt me. I have put in your Ice Age DVD and have some yummy apples for you. When I am done on the phone, I will certainly come to cuddle as well as relax with you!"

If you understand that your child often tends to act out when he/she is tired or hungry, make sure that he/she has enough treats and gets a great night's rest.

Pay attention to your child.

Excellent communication is the most critical tool in your parenting toolbox. When your child misbehaves, put in the time to ask your child what took place, as well as listen to her when he/she describes.

Say your son/daughter has struck his/her good friend. Ask him/her about what happened. You might uncover that he/she hit his/her friend because the close friend would not share a toy, or because he/she is starving or tired and unable to express those feelings suitably.

Restate what your child has informed you. It is an energetic listening technique, as well as modeling it for your children, which will undoubtedly assist their communication skills. For instance, you could say, "I'm hearing you state that you felt mad that your friend would not share. Is that right?"

Speak to your children concerning their feelings.

As soon as you have listened, seize the time to mention areas for development in your child's actions.

You could tell your son/daughter, "You were feeling upset since your buddy wouldn't share. It isn't enjoyable to feel dismayed, is it?" When he/she agrees, you can adhere to up with "When you hit your close friend, it made him/her feel distressed, as well. Do you believe he/she likes feeling disturbed?" This sort of dialogue will encourage your child to consider how others feel and the consequences of his/her actions.

Make a plan for the following time your child feels this way.

It's essential to assist your children in making a plan for what to do when they experience feelings that disturb them and also could result in acting out. This type of action plan is typically utilized for children with ADHD, but it's an excellent idea for all children. You and your son/daughter might come up with a plan that consists of the following steps for the next time he/she feels upset:

- Take a few deep breaths.
- Spend time in another room to cool down.
- Describe what made him/her troubled.

Work out the remedy to his/her issue with moms and dad or in between his/her brother or sister or good friends.

Discuss why you have guidelines.

Frequently, children will act out because they don't understand why they are meant to comply with the policies and expectations you have established.

Clarify to your child specifically why he/she has to adhere to the system you have developed him/her.

For instance, if your son/daughter tosses his/her toys about, you could tell him/her: "We have a guideline that you can't toss your playthings. Throwing your toys could damage them or hurt somebody. It's unsafe, which's why you are not allowed to do it."

Attempt advising your child concerning the "why" the very first time or two he/she breaks the policy. For instance, if you see your son/daughter throwing his/her plaything, ask him/her, "Why do we have the regulation about not tossing playthings?" It will motivate him/her to keep in mind why he/she is not allowed to throw toys.

Follow through and do not give vacant guarantees.

Following up with your words and satisfying your assurances starts to establish count on as well as regard for you as a parent. If you tell your child you will certainly cuddle with him/her, make sure to do so. Otherwise, your child will not trust you and will be more likely to act out and also "call your bluff."

Children are smart as well as will certainly remember what you say. They will certainly likewise attempt to press the limits. You have to remain true to your sentences as well as established limitations for your children.

You likewise have to follow through when you are correcting negative behaviors. If you inform your child that you will undoubtedly remove his/her playthings if he continues to toss them, after that, be sure to take them away if the proceeds of the imperfect action, regardless of your child's unavoidable protests.

Encourage your children by providing options.

Attempt offering the power to your child by giving him/her options in a circumstance. Be strategic in the choices you supply him/her by making both alternatives appropriate habits. For example, claim something like, "You can either get dressed for school now or eat breakfast first." In either case, they are doing what you want in a way you consider acceptable.

Attempt offering your children severe choices that give them no selection but to act. "You can pick to remain here with your good friend yet share and also be good, or you can choose to leave." By doing this, the child is compelled to behave well if he/she intends to remain to have fun.

Show favorable actions instead of negative ones to get the same result.

Your child is likely tossing toys while you get on a phone call to obtain focus. If you educate your child to ask well instead and wait patiently for attention, he will undoubtedly achieve the same result while acting suitably.

If you are asking your child to wait a few more minutes before he/she will undoubtedly get interested. Try making use of a timer to give both of you a concrete concept of the length of time till the child gets what you guaranteed.

Award Good Behavior.

Children look for and also require attention and will undoubtedly seek it in both positive as well as negative ways. Providing positive support aids your child to learn what they are doing well and makes them intend to duplicate that etiquette.

Be very confident in your applauds, by stating things like "Great job cleansing your area as I asked. Thank you!" or "That was fantastic how you shared your toys with your close friends." Or, you can additionally attempt subtle favorable support with smiles, responds, and also hugs.

Producing Effective Consequences

Set out the effects of harmful habits up-front.

When you describe your assumptions for good behavior, additionally explains the consequences for disobeying the expectation. By doing this, your child can choose precisely how to act while understanding what will happen. Say something like, "I anticipate you to hold my hand when we cross the street, and if you do not, you will have to spend ten minutes in time-out." It will make your child to believe even more deeply before he/she takes part in harmful behaviors.

Make each repercussion short as well as easy to understand to raise the chance of your child remembering them. For example, "No iPad today," "No Sesame Street today," or "30 minutes deducted from your computer time today."

Discuss why your child is receiving an consequence.

When you implement a repercussion, make sure your child recognizes why he/she is being penalized. Plainly describe to him/her that you have talked about with him/her what is anticipated, he/she disobeyed you, so now he/she needs to deal with the repercussion. By clearly discussing the consequences, there is no area for complications concerning what behavior was wrong, as well as you will both be on the same page.

Attempt stating something like, "We both concurred that you would certainly not hit other children when they do not share their playthings. Because you hit your close friend, you will certainly not get to play your computer game tonight."

Deal A Choice Of Tangible Rewards When Your Child Engages In Desired Behavior.

Favorable reinforcement is the most positive consequence. When your child behaves in a way that you approve, use him/her an item of candy, and added 10 mins on the playground, or a sticker label.

You can attempt "huge" rewards if your child is exceptionally well behaved for an extensive amount of time, such as having a sleepover, getting ice cream or choosing one thing from the toy store.

Reward, yet do not reward! Rewarding occurs after a behavior is a total, while allurements arise before the truth. If you are approaching your child to act well, he/she may come to be baffled and also think he/she needs to function well when he/she makes money.

Ensure your benefit suits the habits. Using a sticker for sitting through the church silently is acceptable. Yet offering a sticker label for not hitting a classmate could not be a grand adequate incentive. Adopt and adapt to each situation.

Make repercussions short of optimizing their performance.

Children can typically be absent-minded as well as a result, if you make a specific effect last also long, they may fail to remember why they are being punished. If you take your child's toys away since he/she was throwing them, do so just for a few hours or a day, not for a week or a month.

Furthermore, long-term consequences might bring about increased negative habits. For instance, if you ground your child for two months, he might think, "Why should I act? I'm currently grounded."

Always attempt talking to your child first to discover what is going on. Punishment should be used as a last option.

Be consistent.

Picking to establish consequences when it is hassle-free for you is confusing as well as undermines your authority as a parent. By not corresponding, your child may likewise become confused regarding when poor actions will undoubtedly be faced with an effect, and also this will likely cause aggravated behaviors.

HOW TO DISCOVER THE VERY BEST THERAPY FOR YOUR CHILD

Behavior modification is a reliable therapy for attention-deficit/hyperactivity disorder (ADHD) that can improve a child's habits, self-control, and self-confidence. It is most accurate in children when moms and dads supply it. Specialists recommend that doctors refer moms and dads of children more youthful than 12 years of age for training in behavior therapy. For children younger than six years of age, parent training in behavior monitoring should be attempted before prescribing ADHD medicine.

When moms and dads become knowledgeable of behavior modification, they discover skills as well as methods to assist their child with ADHD to do well at school, in your home, and also in relationships. Understanding and practicing behavior therapy requires time and effort. However, it has enduring advantages for the child and the family members.

Did you know?
Parent training in habits administration is likewise called moms and dad behavior therapy, behavioral moms and dad training, or only parent training.

What should parents seek?
Preferably, family members ought to look for a specialist who focuses on training parents. Some specialists will have training or accreditation in moms and dad training program that has been confirmed to work in young children with ADHD.

Therapists may likewise utilize techniques like those in proven programs. The following listing of concerns can be used to find a specialist that utilizes a proven method:

Does this therapist
- Teach moms and dads skills as well as techniques that use favorable support, framework, as well as a convenient routine to manage their child's habits?
- Show parents favorable methods to communicate and interact with their children?
- Appoint activities for parents to exercise with their children?

- Meet regularly with the family to monitor development and also supply mentoring and support?
- Re-evaluate therapy plans, as well as stay adaptable adequate to change strategies as needed?

What can parents expect?

Parents usually participate in eight or even more sessions with a therapist. Sessions might involve dealing with groups of moms and dads or with one family member alone. The therapist meets regularly with the moms and dads to assess their development, offer assistance, and readjust strategies, as required, to ensure transformation. Parents typically practice with their child between sessions.

Parents have the best impact on their child's behavior. Just treatment that focuses on training moms and dads is suggested for children with ADHD because children are not mature enough to transform their habits without their parents' aid. Some therapists might make use of play therapy or talk therapy to treat children with ADHD. Play treatment offers a way for children to communicate their experiences and also sensations through play. Talk therapy utilizes verbal communication in between the child and even a specialist to treat mental and mental illness. Neither of these has been shown to enhance symptoms in children with ADHD.

Learning and also practicing behavior modification requires time and effort, but it has long-lasting advantages for the child. Ask your doctor about the benefits of moms and dad training in behavior modification for young children with ADHD.

What can healthcare providers do?
Doctors can:

- Follow the scientific practice standard for medical diagnosis and therapy of ADHD in young children and external signs
- Review with parents the benefits of behavior therapy as well as why they ought to take into consideration getting training.
- Recognize parent training service providers in their location and also refer moms and dads of young children with ADHD for training in behavior modification before suggesting medicine.

TREATING YOUR CHILD'S ADHD

Observe difficulties with focus. There two types of ADHD signs. For children under 17, a minimum of six of these must exist for an ADHD diagnosis. For older individuals, only five are needed — the first collection of signs associated with issues with focus or attention.

They include:

- Making negligent errors, being unobserving to information
- Having a problem focusing (tasks, playing).
- They are not seeming to listen when a person is talking.
- Not following up on homework, chores, or work, conveniently averted.
- It is organizationally tested.
- Avoiding jobs needing continual focus.
- Not tracking or commonly losing products such as keys, glasses, and so on
- Being conveniently sidetracked.
- Frequently forgetting things.

Hyperactivity.

Theother group ADHD symptoms associated with hyperactivity or absence of impulse control;

Expect the following:

- Fidgeting or agonizing; tapping hands or feet.
- Feeling troubled, running, or climbing up inappropriately.
- Having a hard time to remain quiet.
- Speaking exceedingly.
- They are spouting out answers before inquiries are asked.
- Having a hard time to await his/her turn.
- Disturbing others.

Discover the causes of ADHD.

The brain of an individual with ADHD is somewhat different than others. Two frameworks specifically tend to be smaller sized: the basal ganglia and the prefrontal cortex.

The first ganglia regulate the motion of muscular tissues.

It indicates which must be working as well as which must be at rest at any given time.

If a child is resting at a work desk in the classroom, the first ganglia needs to send out a message informing the feet to remain still. In the case of ADHD, the feet may not obtain the news. They may stay in motion. A shortage of the first ganglia can likewise often cause fidgety hand motions. For example, individuals with ADHD might tap a pencil on a desk or drum their fingers.

The prefrontal cortex is essential for conducting higher-order jobs.

It is where memory, discovering, and focusing come together. This area is necessary for intellectual features.

The prefrontal cortex plays an essential function in managing natural chemical dopamine.

Dopamine influences your ability to focus and usually is at reduced degrees in persons with ADHD.

Serotonin is one more neurotransmitter related to the prefrontal cortex. It affects mood, rest, and also appetite. When serotonin drops as well lessens, clinical depression as well as stress and anxiety result.

Lower degrees of dopamine and serotonin can make it harder to focus. Because of this, individuals with ADHD struggle to concentrate on one thing at a time and are more easily sidetracked.

Look out for relevant problems.

ADHD commonly occurs together with various other mental health issues. It is called "comorbidity."

One in five individuals with ADHD likewise has some other significant disorder. Depression and bipolar affective disorder are the most common.

One in threechildren with ADHD also has a behavior condition. These include conduct problems as well as different defiance conditions.

Learning disabilities and also anxiousness likewise generally appear along with ADHD.

See a medical professional for medical diagnosis.

If you or a loved one has many of these traits, you need to see a doctor to get an expert point of view. Understanding if ADHD might be the reason for these troubles will certainly help you pick the best therapy.

Dealing with ADHD

Obtain a prescription for the right drug.

For most individuals with ADHD, medication is a fundamental part of therapy. There are two classifications of ADHD medication: stimulants (such as methylphenidate as well as amphetamine) and also non-stimulants (such as guanfacine as well as atomoxetine).

Using stimulants to treat ADHD may not seem like it makes much feeling.

The components of the mind they stimulate, however, are accountable for impulse control and also focus. Energizers like Ritalin, Concerta, and also Adderall can assist in regulating neurotransmitters like norepinephrine and also dopamine.

Non-stimulant anti-depression drugs frequently used to treat ADHD manage the same neurotransmitters. They do so through a different chemical procedure. Doctors might recommend them if stimulants don't work or have rough side-effects.

Choosing the best medication can be tough.

Different individuals respond in different ways to different medications. The performance of some medicines can also transform throughout development surges, hormone fluctuations, diet plan as well as weight modifications, and with the flow of time. The best method to choose the ideal medicine is through discussion with your doctor. Bear in mind that if something does not seem to be functioning, you can speak to your medical professional concerning attempting a different choice.

Some medicines are available in extended-release varieties. They launch active ingredients progressively over the day. It removes the demand to take extra dosages at school or work.

Eat a diet regimen that combats ADHD.

Some foods can lower the effects of the hormonal shortages that are usually component of ADHD. Here are some suggestions.

Complex carbohydrates can raise serotonin degrees. It can suggest a better mood, sleep, and also appetite. Attempt to consume foods like whole grains, eco-friendly vegetables, starchy vegetables, and even beans. These foods release energy progressively. Avoid necessary carbs like sugars, honey, jelly, candy, soft drink, and so on. These can create a temporary serotonin spike, yet do more injury than great over the future.

A diet plan abundant in healthy protein can boost focus. Try to include numerous healthy proteins throughout the day to keep dopamine degrees high. Great sources of protein consist of meat, fish, nuts, legumes, and beans.

Take zinc. Zinc advertises to lower degrees of attention deficit disorder as well as impulsivity. Consume seafood, fowl strengthened grains as well as various other foods with a high zinc web content and take zinc supplements.

Eating specific spices might also assist. Saffron may counter clinical depression, while cinnamon can aid with interest and also focus.

Stay clear of foods that worsen ADHD.

Various other foods can sometimes make the problem worse.

Stay clear of "negative fats" such as trans fats and those discovered in fried foods, burgers, and pizza. Select foods high in omega-3 fatty acids rather. Excellent sources include salmon, walnuts, as well as avocados. These might assist reduced hyperactivity as well as enhance coping skills.

Prevent food with dyes and also food coloring. Some studies suggest there may be a web link between food dyes and ADHD signs and symptoms. The red color, in particular, might be a problem.

Minimize consumption of wheat as well as dairy products, sugar, refined foods, and additives. These foods might negatively affect ADHD signs.

Obtain treatment for ADHD.

A good therapist can help you and your loved ones handle the challenges of ADHD. Treatment usually starts by analyzing the family members' structure. The therapist will certainly typically recommend changes to create an environment that deals with the mind functions of a person with ADHD.

Treatment also offers a refuge for family members to vent their irritations in a healthy and balanced means. It is a venue to work out concerns with specialist support.

Experts commonly recommend that young children with ADHD obtain behavioral therapy. This approach educates people on exactly how to change behavior and control impulses.

Adults with ADHD usually take advantage of psychotherapy. It aids them to accept who they are while looking for renovations to their circumstances.

Individuals with ADHD gain significantly from discovering more about their problems. Therapy aids them to comprehend that they are not alone in their struggles.

Get plenty of exercise.

Exercise stimulates the production of much of the same neurotransmitters as ADHD medication. Extreme workouts are a fantastic way to manage your brain chemistry, but also a couple of 30 minutes strolls every week can make a huge difference.

Specifically, exercise promotes the production of dopamine, norepinephrine, and also serotonin. All these can assist boost focus and attention.

Utilizing Everyday Strategies For Coping.

Arrange the environment.

People with ADHD are continually trying to understand their settings. Organizing the residence is a fantastic method to begin.

People with ADHD frequently have difficulty bearing in mind where they put things. Having assigned containers, tubs, shelves, or hooks for different sorts of products can make life much more comfortable.

It is especially essential for children, that gain from well-organized bedrooms and also play locations.

Assist children to remain organized by supplying color-coded containers as well as bathtubs. You can also identify these with photos or words explaining the types of items that belong within.

Similar business strategies can additionally benefit adults in the workplace.

Decrease distractions.

People with ADHD additionally have trouble filtering out disturbances in the environment. Below are a few pointers for lowering interruptions in the home or office.

Switch off the TV and stereo when you are not watching or listening. Both of these can be distracting. It is especially important when an individual with ADHD is trying to concentrate or when you are attempting to interact with children.

Readjust lights. Lighting that creates shadows or unique patterns can be distracting for individuals with ADHD. Make lights in your home regularly, and change flickering light bulbs right away. Stay away from fluorescent illumination, as the hum of the bulbs can likewise make it challenging to focus.

Avoid strong scents. Distinctive smells can likewise make it hard for someone with ADHD to focus. Prevent aromatic air fresheners, as well as fragrances as well as colognes.

Establish a routine.

People with ADHD succeed with constant routines. Doing the very same thing at the very same time and also in the same place, each day makes it easier to bear in mind and also concentrate on essential jobs.

For children, having a particular time allotted for homework and also tasks is helpful. It can additionally reduce disagreements around these topics.

Breaking routine tasks down into small, convenient pieces likewise assists. Individuals with ADHD have a problem holding great deals of instructions in their heads at the very same time. Even things that appear simple can be simplified. Filling the dishwasher can be broken up into packing the top rack, lower shelf, and silverware.

For young people with ADHD, appreciation and also little incentives at each action can aid enhance the pattern. For deviations, instant, as well as a regular discipline, can additionally help. Make sure the effects of wrongdoing coincide every time and also come swiftly after the actions.

Developing a framework throughout school breaks is specifically crucial for children and teenagers. Urge them to sign up with assigned tasks that have standard conferences. Examples include summertime supply plays, sports groups, or clubs.

Utilize a planner.

Keeping a planner or schedule can be useful for people with ADHD. It can be a place to record the everyday routine, along with details jobs like homework or work conferences.

A planner is most handy if you inspect and upgrade it often.

You can use applications or on-line planners with visible or audible suggestions to make sure you do not forget visits or set up jobs.

For children, it is a great idea to ask teachers to review the planner every day to make sure the pupil has recorded homework correctly.

Looking For Help in School or the Workplace.

Obtain assistance in school. Schools supply numerous services for children with ADHD.

These services range from extra time on tests to self-supporting classes with specially trained teachers and aides.

Interact with educators to make sure they understand the nature of the child's condition. Some educators mistake ADHD for stubbornness or an attitude problem.

Ask for individual education evaluation. It will allow you to work with the school to produce an Individual Education Plan (IEP) for the student. This document specifies goals for the pupil, along with interventions and also strategies for getting to those goals. Make sure to send the assessment request before creating one.

You'll produce an IEP with school officials. Do not permit the school to pressure you right into signing a "one-size-fits-all" IEP. It needs to be customized to the needs of the individual student.

Get a help-seeking job.

There are additionally service offered for people with ADHD that are looking for employment. These are provided by schools, state companies, and also non-profit organizations.

A variety of transitional solutions are readily available to aid school-aged children to apply for school, professional school, or jobs. It includes help with filling out applications, talking to, and also independent living. Transitional solutions must be the focus of IEPs for pupils over the age of 16.

All states in the US deal with employment rehab (VR) services. These are services for individuals with disabilities who need aid looking for or keeping work. Virtual Reality therapists can sometimes help with financial help to a university or vocational training camp. For instance, a VR program could sponsor truck-driving classes to obtain an industrial driver's permit. Search your state federal government's website to see what solutions are available.

Other Virtual Reality services may include the computer of job abilities training. A Virtual Reality program may supply hearing aids or various other flexible modern technology. It may also provide help completing applications or producing resumes and practicing interviewing abilities.

Obtain help in maintaining work. People with ADHD often battle to keep on tasks.

Issues with focus, time administration, and also, in some cases, social abilities create obstacles to rewarding work. Here are a few suggestions for getting help.

Connect with managers and coworkers concerning the limitations that feature ADHD. If they discover the problem, they are most likely to be thoughtful as well as consider it.

Virtual Reality solutions additionally offer training that can make it simpler to function at the office. They can help with work abilities as well as the organization. Again, examine the state's website to see what solutions are readily available.

You can employ a task coach that will undoubtedly go through your workday with you. He or she will search for issues as well as make recommendations to you and also your employer for making your work extra efficient and even productive. Virtual Reality solutions typically offer or spend on task mentoring. Charitable organizations in your area might likewise provide this service.

RESOURCES FOR PARENTS AS WELL AS CHILDREN WITH ADHD

Resources for ADHD

Attention deficit disorder (ADHD) is just one of the most typical childhood neurodevelopmental conditions. It affects as much as five percent of children in the United States.

According to the American Psychiatric Association (APA), approximately 2.5 percent of adults likewise deal with this condition. Men are three times most likely to be diagnosed with ADHD than females.

Children, as well as adults with ADHD, might deal with impulse control, hyperactivity, as well as problems paying attention for extended periods. Left neglected, it can interrupt one's capability to process, comprehend, as well as discover details.

Numerous sources and treatments – such as medication and behavioral therapy – can assist those with ADHD who live satisfying and useful lives. There are additionally a variety of organizations, resources, and also academic devices – like the ones listed below – that can aid those with ADHD and their friends and family.

Not-for-profit companies

Nonprofit companies can be a practical resource, using valuable info regarding ADHD, along with info for friends and family members.

Below are companies that supply sources for children, as well as adults coping with ADHD Not-for-profit organizations found in Canada as well as the United Kingdom, are also consisted of.

- CHADD: The National Resource for ADHD.
- Attention Deficit Disorder Association (ADDA).
- Centre for ADHD Awareness, Canada (CADDAC).
- ADHD Foundation: Mental Health, Education, and Training Services.
- The American Professional Society of ADHD as well as Related Disorders.
- ADHD World Federation: Child and Adult Disorder.
- Child Mind Institute.

SETTING ROUTINES/HABITS FOR A CHILD WITH ADHD

Children with ADHD need routine. Trusted schedules for mornings, after school, and bedtime make an incredible distinction in establishing expectations, building desirable behaviors, as well as improving ADD-related habits. Utilize these suggested layouts to dispute your family members' time.

All parents of children with ADHD have listened to the routine concerning routines: Children require a framework, as well as children with attention-deficit, require a lot more. The keys to getting the ADHD company aid you need: idea in the power of family regimens and also a lasting dedication to them.

You've heard it before: set up an early morning routine for children with ADHD to go out the door on time. Make sure research happens at the same time as well as in the very same setting daily. Do something fun to loosen up before a regular bedtime.

Theoretically, this appears pretty necessary. When you're raising a child with actual focus troubles in the real world, establishing and keeping such routines can seem downright helpless. Yet there is hope – also a joy – insight.

Many sympathetic moms and dads enthusiastically start to establish the structure their children require. Yet lots of surrender after a couple of weeks (or even a few days) because the regimens are not functioning. "Billy will not listen. He does not wish to follow it. Each day comes to be a fight, and we're all worn. Is there another thing we can try?"

Usually, trying to execute a daily routine doesn't function since parents give up prematurely. To make structure genuinely reliable, regimens require to be seen as well as implemented not equally as basic behavioral techniques; however, as a way of living.

The Benefits of placing Your Child on a Schedule

Regimens impact life favorably on two levels. In regards to habits, they help enhance performance and daily functioning. It may not always be apparent, but children want as well as require routines. A foreseeable method offers a structure that helps children feel safe and secure. By developing one, you send out a message that states, "This is how we do things." Routines make everyday tasks convenient, allowing your child to focus on one thing at a time.

Additionally, your entire family will benefit mentally from a structured regimen. Both parents and children experience lowered stress when there's much less dramatization regarding what time you'll eat supper and also where you'll calm down to do homework.

What follows is a relaxed residence, which generates stronger family partnerships. And also, family member's identification is solidified by routines in which every person contributes (Anna sets the table, Brian clears the meals). The message: we are relatives who eat together; we are family members that read with each other; we are a family who routines standard times for schoolwork and also other ongoing responsibilities.

In these desperate times, it might appear challenging to give a structured way of life. Every person is juggling timetables: job, school, entertainment, music lessons, basketball technique, and so on. Yet in just such times, the structure ends up being crucial. The benefit: higher productivity for your child, in addition to better wellness and also household relationships.

A review of 50 years of psychological research study, just recently released in the Journal of Family Psychology, shows that even infants, as well as young children, are healthier and display better-regulated habits when there are predictable routines in the household.

Effective regimens take commitment as well as consistency, with all family members adults providing a united front. Regimens should be developed when children are young and used continuously as they grow – but it's never too late to begin. Above all, don't quit.

Here are suggestions and some example routines to begin with. You'll want to modify them to match the age as well as the maturation of your child, the specific actions you are working on, as well as your family's character as well as needs. As you establish your regimens, bear in mind that success takes some time – often months and also years. Yet the benefits will undoubtedly last a lifetime.

Greetings Start with Your Child's Schedule

The objective of the early morning routine is to obtain every person all set and also out the door on time. Preparations made the night before, such as showering, loading book bags, outlining clothing, setting the alarm, and creating lunch, are essential in establishing a smooth morning routine.

Since lots of children (and adults) with ADHD are very distractible and also spontaneous, prevent stimuli that are likely to get focus as well as toss the routine of the training course. Some tips include:

- Leave the TV off in the early morning.
- Do not hop on the computer system to check your e-mails.
- Neglect that brand-new magazine or directory till after school or later that night.

After School Schedule: Homework Helpers

It's frequently stated that the only constant thing about children with ADHD is their disparity. This is particularly problematic when it involves academic effort. No activity demands a more significant structure and also uniformity than homework when a child's capability to self-regulate is called upon. Not surprisingly, parent-child homework battles are frequent. Yet a well-known study routine (time, place, approaches) goes a lengthy method toward lowering their frequency and also strength – otherwise eliminating them. To develop a homework routine that will certainly enhance efficiency as well as boost scholastic success:

1. Impose a regular begin time. It will assist your child in developing a research behavior.

2. Stay near to your child. Lots of children with ADHD concentrate much better when an adult work with them or neighbors.
3. Take breaks. Distractibility, uneasiness, trouble maintaining concentration, and also reduced irritation tolerance – all common of ADHD – practically guarantee psychological fatigue and monotony. Regular time-outs, during which the child is permitted to move, can aid.
4. Have a good time afterward. Your child is most likely to use herself to research when she knows that fun activity, such as playing a game or viewing TV, will undoubtedly follow.

A Consistent Dinnertime Schedule

For centuries, families have built solid relationships around the table. In this age of the Internet as well as TV films as needed, a dinner ritual is still useful, if not essential. While most nourishments last only about 20 mins (much less time than a TV comedy), a lot of good ideas can take place in that short time. Preferably, nourishments should be real social time, with business, school, or family problems left off the table. It takes time and also work to prepare a household meal, and also it can be trouble getting everybody together at once. Yet, you'll discover the advantages are well worth the initiative:

Members of the family stay attached to each other's lives.

Occasions are reviewed as well as preparations are made with everybody's input.

Responsibility, as well as family cohesion, are motivated by such easy work as children establishing the table and also tidying up later on.

Great Nights Begin with a Bedtime Routine

Your objective at bedtime is to aid your child wind down and get to rest at a typical time. Study reveals that children with routine bedtime regimens get to relax sooner and also stir up much less usually throughout the night than those without them. Several children with ADHD battle bedtime since, going to sleep is annoying to them. It's time for rest. However, there's still so much they can do! Routines that provide benefits as well as a pleasurable activity while motivating relaxation can aid overcome the monotony of bedtime. Some things to try:

- Have a light, healthy, and balanced snack, like an apple or cheese on a rice cake.
- Play a quiet, low-stakes video game, or read a publication.

- Have a sweet and also individual nighttime lights-out ritual.
- Try to obtain your child right into bed at the same time each night.

No question about it. Developing family routines takes a lot of time and effort. You may ask yourself, "Can we afford the time as well as the energy to do every one of this?" A much better concern might be, "Can we afford not to?

ADHD Organization Help: A Sample Schedule

7:00 a.m. Tickle your child out of bed(a little delighted energy can get her up and also moving quickly).

7:05 a.m. Get all set: Post a listing as well as have your child stick to it.

- Clean face.
- Brush hair.
- Get dressed (clothes are set out the night before). Examine to see how your child is doing but let her comply with the listing and do for herself.

7:20 a.m. Breakfast time: Offer two healthy and balanced yet enticing selections, max. You would like her to spend her time eating, not yearning over Lucky Charms.

7:45 a.m. Brush your teeth – together. Being with her can pace things up and also ensure great hygiene.

7:55 a.m. Zip, connection, and layer up. Keeping shoes and also hand wear covers by the front door saves you the hide-and-seek.

8:00 a.m. Out you go.

Test Homework schedule.

3:00 p.m. Have a cookie and also relax from school.

3:30 p.m. Settle your child at his normal homework area; make sure all devices are offered (pencils, paper, calculator, referral publications, and so on).

3:35 – 4:30 p.m. Your child does homework; you remain around to respond to questions and monitor breaks (stretch, restroom, drink).

4:25 p.m. Check his work, as well as calmly review anything he must modify (however, don't do it for him). Offer details praise job entirely.

Test Dinner schedule.

6:00 p.m. Parents start food preparation. Arrange prep work to make sure that you can stay clear of the delay of nourishment.

6:15 p.m., children set the table. Give them specific tasks to introduce a sense of obligation.

6:30 p.m. Children place the drinks.

6:45 p.m. The mother brings the foodstuff bent on the table.

7:00 p.m. Dinner is offered. For banquet talk, try this: Go around the table – as soon as or more – and also have each person share one good idea concerning the child's day at large

7:30 p.m. Children clear the table. Moms and dad(s) loads the dishwasher.

Experience a Bedtime Routine.

8:00 p.m. Let him unwind in the tub. You can check on him or he can monitor himself. After cleaning, a bathroom can help a child mellow out at day's end.

8:20 p.m. Three-part routine: dry off, brush teeth, as well as pee. You do not want to listen to, "Mom, I have to go to the restroom!" five minutes after you say goodnight.

8:30 p.m. Get right into PJs and clean up toys to establish nighttime, not a play, situation.

8:40 p.m. Read together.

8:55 p.m. Your child gets into bed. Do your nighttime custom: talk a little about the day, praise your child on the things he succeeded, claim your ritual goodnight – "I like you right to the moon as well as back again. Do not let the bug bite."

MEDICATIONS COMMONLY PRESCRIBED FOR ADHD

1. Methylphenidates: This household of energizers is utilized to treat both ADHD and narcolepsy. Trademark name are: Ritalin, Concerta, Metadate, Focalin, Daytrana

2. Dextroamphetamine: brand names are Exedrine, Vyvanse.

3. Amphetamines: These medications were as soon as accepted by the FDA in the 1960s for the therapy of weight problems as well as ADHD. One of the most typical brands is Adderall.

Ritalin, Concerta, Metadate, Focalin, Daytrana.

Medication bottle Ritalin, methylphenidate, is the most commonly recommended medication for ADHD. The first proposed dose is 5 mg of the short-acting range for young children, as well as 10 mg for older children, teenagers, and also adults. The majority of people take a morning and even a lunch dosage. Some people also need a mid-afternoon dose to finish homework or various other required tasks. Clients (and caretakers) are encouraged to track action to medication and also record back to the recommending doctor. If adverse effects are marginal, the company will progressively increase the dose until the person notices enhancement. Children, as well as their caregivers, must not boost the treatment without talking to their doctor. The maximum advised dosage of Ritalin is 60 mg per day. This higher dosage usually is tried before switching to various medications.

If Ritalin is active, and an optimum dose has been determined, the service provider may recommend switching over to long-acting (LA) formula. It gets rid of the need for greater than one dosage each day. Ritalin LA is created with a 50% prompt release, as well as a 50% delayed-release. This two-tiered release prolongs the medicine's performance for approximately eight hours. It generates two equivalent stage does, one in the morning as well as one in the mid-day. It functions well for many individuals, but not all. Locating one of the most effective dosages may call for perseverance and adaptability as various methods are checked.

Focalin is a reliable type of methylphenidate. It has only been approximately for about ten years. Productive medication activity can be beneficial for some adults or enormous individuals. It may be too intense for young children and may also trigger lots of side effects. Focalin can be found in a pill with 50% immediate release, and even 50% postponed the launch. It lasts for12 hours.

Another option is Daytrana, which is a methylphenidate spot. Primarily, the place has medication that's ingrained in the adhesive. You peel the liner, and the adhesive holds it next to the skin. The drug is taken in with the skin, straight into the bloodstream. A patch offers an extra even and steady dose than pills taken in via the intestinal tract track.

Nonetheless, it takes longer to work. Once a therapeutic degree is received, the medication level remains very continuous for about 9 to 10 hours or up until the spot is removed. Blood levels return to standard regarding an hour and a fifty percent after removing the patch.

Dexedrine, Exedrine,

If Ritalin does not show effective, Dexedrine, a Dextroamphetamine, is the following, probably a candidate to try. Concerning 12% of individuals with ADHD are treated with this medication. In addition to influencing dopamine levels, Dexedrine likewise affects norepinephrine degrees. Norepinephrine is an additional natural chemical that affects our capacity to pay attention as well as focus.

This medication decreases tiredness, increases electric motor task and psychological performance, and also produces moderate euphoria. The adverse effects of making use of Dexedrine consist of enhanced heart rate, blood vessel restriction, and bronchial dilation. However, the critical problem regarding its use is connected to its potential to be re-sealed as a road medicine. It is two times as powerful as Ritalin, as well as is highly valued in the underground drug trade.

A 5 mg dose lasts typically five to six hours. Using Dexedrine adds flexibility to a therapy program because there are three strengths of slow-release tablets. These are much more dependable than slow-release Ritalin; they are harder to get because they are a lot more closely monitored by the DEA.

Viviane

Vyvanse is an additional amphetamine; however, it additionally includes a substance called lysine. Lysine affixes itself to the active component in Adderall, an amphetamine. To metabolize this drug, an added action is required to disintegrate Lysine from Adderall. This combined process ensures that Vyvanse lasts a long time-up to 14 hours. Although this length of time can conveniently be also long for a little one, maybe perfect for people in senior high school or university, or a grownup. It's a powdered medication, so it will certainly have a regular launch, without peaks as well as troughs.

Adderall

Adderall is an immediate-acting amphetamine. Its impact will certainly last for three to four hours. Adderall XR (extended-release) is a mix of both prompt and also slow-release forms. The XR type lasts up to 10 to 12 hours (two times as lengthy as Dexedrine). The advantage of the XR type is it generally needs only one dosage per day. Both unbiased efficiency actions (e.g., qualities, tests), as well as subjective measures (e.g., teacher scores), suggest both forms of Adderall work. The adverse effects of Adderall are similar to Dexedrine. The recommended dose for children is five to 60 mg. This broad range suggests the different reactions of private children as an outcome of dimension, metabolism, and also the age of the child.

National Drug Administration is a company in the United States in charge of drug guidelines. In 2005, the FDA launched a warning about making use of Adderall in response to 12 pediatric deaths. With further examination, extenuating scenarios were found in each situation. These consisted of heat

197

exhaustion, Type I diabetes, dehydration, as well as incredibly vigorous exercise. Some children had hidden heart conditions that added to their fatality. The FDA compared the rate of premature death for these cases of pediatric Adderall individuals, versus the early death rate in the general pediatric populace. This comparison revealed comparable rates.

Consequently, the FDA is remaining to explore the connection between Adderall as well as sudden death. Nonetheless, the FDA has not removed Adderall from the marketplace. Currently, there are no more limitations on Adderall, other than a warning that individuals with underlying heart disease are at particular danger.

COMPARING DRUGS FOR ADHD

	Stimulants	Non-Stimulants: Atomoxetine (Strattera) as well as Alpha-2 Adrenergics
The Way Or Manner They Work	Generally, target receptors of the brain chemical	Atomoxetine (Strattera): Targets the brain chemical

	dopamine.	norepinephrine. It can develop attention and reduce impulsivity and hyperactivity.
	Very efficient at improving alertness and reducing hyperactivity and impulsivity	Alpha-2 adrenergic: How they operate in the brain to assist with ADHD is unclear. However, they minimize attention deficit disorder and impulsivity. They might likewise boost interest.
How rapidly They Start And Stop Working	Fast performing. A child will feel results within 30 to 90 minutes of the very first dosage, depending upon the medicine as well as individual sensitivity.	Atomoxetine (Strattera): Takes two to four weeks for the drug to have complete results. Children can be reduced swiftly, generally within a few days.

	These drugs – and their impacts – leave the system within three to 12 hours, relying on whether they're short-acting or long-acting.	Alpha-2 adrenergic: Takes two weeks to understand if the medicine works. Children's overdoses over the long-term might require to be lessened gradually to avoid side effects when the drug is stopped.
Dosing Frequency	Extended-release pills last six to 12 hours – adequate to cover the school day	Atomoxetine (Strattera): Once, sometimes two times, a day Alpha-2 adrenergic: From one to three times a day.
Common Side Effects	Loss of appetite, difficulty sleeping (Uncommon adverse effects consist of boosted	Atomoxetine (Strattera): Moodiness. (Uncommon adverse effects include nausea or vomiting,

	stress and anxiety, agitation, frustrations, tics, psychosis).	anorexia nervosa, slowness). Alpha-2 adrenergic: Sleepiness, exhaustion. (Uncommon adverse effects consist of loss of appetite, drop in high blood pressure, queasiness.)
Danger	Could cause weight management and possibly impact elevation. (Weight, as well as height, should be monitored). Use with care in children with pre-existing heart conditions since	Atomoxetine (Strattera): Scarce incidence of liver difficulties. Alpha-2 adrenergic: May cause dizziness as well as passing out if it significantly impacts high blood pressure.

	these medications can, in uncommon instances, create problems. A cardiologist ought to authorize the child taking it.	
Efficiency	It improves interest as well as decreases impulsivity as well as attention deficit disorder in 70 to 80 percent of patients.	Atomoxetine (Strattera): Improves interest and also lowers impulsivity and attention deficit disorder in about 50 percent of patients. Alpha-2 adrenergic: Reduces impulsivity as well as attention deficit disorder in 60 percent of patients.
Doctors Might recommend These Drugs	Generally, this is the first line of medical therapy for children with ADHD and ADD.	Atomoxetine (Strattera): Maybe prescribed if a child can't endure the side effects of stimulants. It may also be an alternative for teens

		as well as young adults that may benefit from 24-hour coverage.
		Alpha-2 adrenergic: Most frequently utilized in addition to stimulants to help children with severe signs.

HELPFUL TIPS FOR RAISING CHILDREN WITH ADHD

Get a little self-centered

Research studies reveal that parental stress may boost when increasing a child with ADHD (mainly when various other conditions are likewise existing), which can result in many more parenting battles down the road.

Sometimes it takes a scientific study with substantial information to remind us that stress, overload, and also exhaustion is real as well as not some imperfection we can will away.

In a world where your child always comes first, you need to schedule in minutes that prioritize you.

Whatever that resembles – a stroll with your canine, kickball with close friends, a foamy cappuccino, krav maga, or a face-first-in-the-pillow nap – trust us when we say focusing on yourself will help you be a better parent.

2. Self-control your child the same, but different

Children with ADHD need a somewhat different method, which suggests you require to be adaptable.

Your pal's child is tossing playthings and battling his teddy bear after recess. Typical parenting code would undoubtedly consider this time-out deserving. It's the very same for children with ADHD, however not.

Since hyperactivity is a sign and symptom of ADHD, this behavior is often an outcome of their problem. It doesn't mean that they feel untouchable – you require to select the proper penalty and also strategy.

Yelling at a child for their ADHD-related actions does not help them create the abilities they need to self-regulate, as well as they might wind up acting out much more if they feel they'll get argued with regardless.

Attempt penalties, like a break, that feel routine, structured, and also give clear guidelines regarding why the habits aren't alright.

3. Produce as well as stick to a routine

Regimens are your child's buddy now.

You do not need to box them in with regulations on guidelines, but many children with ADHD thrive under an established routine since they haven't found out how to prioritize things on their own.

It mainly applies to your routines before and after school.

While walking away is most important, you can increase on that organizing power by hanging a complete schedule someplace prominent in your house, like the kitchen.

Track your family members' to-do's, visits, and vital things to remember. If your child is mature enough for a tablet, phone, or computer system, try establishing digital pointers as well as signals.

Not only will your child feel concentrated as well as support, yet it'll keep you responsible, also.

4. Establish clear guideline – and also really follow them

Remember our talk about routines? It also applies to fundamental rules in your home.

It helps to reduce complications your child could have regarding actions, such as leaving the table throughout mealtimes. You can even ask your child to help set a few of these policies once they're old enough.

5. Take things one step at a time

Taking it slow can teach your child a more important lesson: mindfulness.

Sure, it seems chic; however, in addition to various other advantages, science has located mindfulness to be efficient at minimizing ADHD signs and symptoms.

By selecting a simple job, like placing books back on a shelf, and persevering from start to finish, you help your teen exercise their very own ability to concentrate.

Avoid giving them numerous tasks at a time, as well as do your best to be a support.

6. Focus on play and also exercise

There's boosting proof that exercise can help children with ADHD.

By advertising neural development as well as cognitive development, researches recommend that getting your children proceeding a regular basis might help minimize some of their signs and symptoms.

You'll establish them up for a healthy and balanced, active life.

7. Make food prep ADHD-friendly

While there's no definitive study, numerous parents discover that sticking to particular dietary limitations can help alleviate some of their child's ADHD signs.

A healthy and balanced diet regimen consisting of fresh vegetables and fruits, whole grains, as well as lean proteins is good for everybody.

However, parents might likewise take into consideration removing or reducing certain foods and components, consisting of yet not restricted to sugary foods and ones with artificial shades as well as chemicals.

You can also try adding more omega-3 fats – also known as fish, nuts, and even seeds.

8. Perfect the art of the kickback

Okay, so you're not the God Father, yet incentivizing tasks will certainly produce a positive organization with cleansing, something several children with ADHD deal with.

If you've ever before explained your child's space as looking like a bomb went off, you understand what we indicate below.

To keep that room tidy, you require to initial lead by instance.

Do your best to keep things at home clean, in spite of how appealing it is to let the recipes soak for another two days. Then, draw out the kickbacks incentives.

Ideally, these won't impact your child's routines, so try things like allowing them to select the after-dinner movie or a factors system that adds up to a new toy, publication, or item of clothes.

9. Make going to bed a special event

You don't need us to tell you that sleep is essential for growing children, yet it bears repeating: Sleep is so crucial for your child's growth and administration of their ADHD.

The trouble? Children with ADHD are susceptible to rest concerns, especially if they are taking medication for their condition. To battle this, focus on healthy sleep patterns for your family.

That consists of having a set time for going to bed, possibly offering melatonin (ask your doc regarding how to do this properly) and switching off screens about a half hour before bed.

10. When unsure, try behavior therapy

Ask your pediatrician to connect you with a therapist who can educate you about behavior therapy.

Because moms and dads have such a substantial impact on their children, it is most useful that children get their therapy directly from them.

A few sessions with an expert will reveal to you how to give positive interaction, positive support, framework, and also discipline for your child.

11. If you have an older child, do not hesitate to let them in on the action

Every parent loves the day their infant ends up being a teen, as well as World War III, erupts in their house.

Reality 1: This occurs to everybody, as well as you're not alone.

Reality 2: ADHD makes this turmoil even more challenging to browse, both for you and your child.

Enter behavior modification 2.0. For children in middle school and also senior high school, a specialist could be the very best individual to help them navigate their signs and symptoms.

This type of therapy delivered by a neutral third party can be specifically practical for children presenting defiance and also resistance (which is basically what teen roadways are led with).

Ask your doctor for a specialist recommendation. Not only can they help your teen, however, but they'll also have plenty of tips for maintaining an open discussion about treatment and ways to show judgment-free support.

12. Speak with your child's teachers, but don't be a "helicopter" moms and dad

Teachers spend concerning seven hours a day with your children at school. Shouldn't you give them all the means to make the most of those hours?

First things first, talk with your child's educators and care providers about your child's diagnosis. Probabilities are this isn't their very first rodeo, and also, they'll recognize how to continue.

Enter prepared to answer inquiries as well as offer descriptions, yet do not turn the meeting into an hour-long ADHD 101 program.

The objective is to allow any individual caring for your child to leave with an understanding of how to stay up to date with well-established regimens, recognize triggers, and also make a plan to help your child flourish.

Maintain having these conversations frequently so that everyone stays on the same page. Your child's teacher could even have fresh ADHD parenting ideas from their very own communications with your child.

13. For extra support in school, consider an IEP or Section 504

When the traditional educational program isn't sufficing, conversation with your child's school concerning producing an Independent Education Plan.

If they are not qualified for an IEP, you might still have the ability to obtain help using Section 504, which needs schools to supply assistance to learners with learning specials needs.

Keep in mind that you'll need a diagnosis from your child's doctor in advance.

Additionally, be honest with your child before making the change. No person wants to be selected as different in school, yet if your little one is battling, a tailored understanding plan can be what they need.

14. Let them fidget

Some children focus far better when they have an outlet for their fidgeting. You've become aware of fidget rewriters, but there's, in fact, a vast world of fantastic fidget-friendly playthings available.

Offering your child an outlet throughout moments when they're asked to sit still can help them concentrate much better in your home and at school (after you check with their teacher, obviously).

15. Demand designated seats

We understand we said not to be a helicopter mom and dad, but in this instance, going the extra mile can be valuable. An ADHD learner's seat should be purposefully put within a classroom.

Deal with their teacher to locate an appropriate area, such as near the instructor, near the front of the classroom, or away from way too many distractions.

16. Take your child to yoga exercise

Whether you take part with each other or sign them up for a children's yoga group.

A regular yoga exercise practice has been revealed to lower symptoms of ADHD and has generally been confirmed efficient for dealing with issues like nervousness and anxiety.

17. Try out vital oils

The science is still mediocre right here, as well as it's certainly not a substitute for legit therapies like behavior therapy. Yet, necessary oils are one more path numerous parents of children with ADHD speak highly of.

Oils like rosemary, peppermint, and lavender have actually all been connected to leisure and boosted concentration. Attempt establishing a diffuser while your child does homework or including a few drops to their bathroom water.

Just be cautious to prevent contact with eyes, as well as do not apply to skin without diluting in the water or oil.

18. Make technology your close friend

As a parent, it's just natural to have made complicated feelings concerning play time. Still, if they're going to have electronic devices, you could as well utilize the sources available on them.

Younger children will benefit from you taking the lead in assisting them to remain organized with their research, jobs, and also extracurriculars.

Yet older teenagers can take advantage of making use of these on their own to track tasks, part-time work schedules, university exams, study sessions, athletic contests, and also a lot more.

19. Look inside their head

Ever before, wish you could know what's taking place inside your child's head? Some individuals have discovered success in treating ADHD symptoms with neuro feedback.

This sort of training permits a child to actually see exactly how their brain responds to the job of focus, and also might help them discover far better tactics for remaining focused.

20. Spend even more time outside

Studies have revealed that time outdoors is beneficial for all, but a lot more so for children with ADHD, who frequently have a much easier time concentrating after investing a little time in nature.

21. Display display time

Pun not meant. A lot more study is needed, however limiting screen time can help maintain ADHD signs and symptoms at bay.

Some researches recommend that children and also teenagers with ADHD are more vulnerable to evaluate dependency problems, so it's best to keep an eye out for extreme phone or computer system use.

Try going for a walk, playing a video game, or exercising a brand-new skill with all that additional free time.

22. Keep an open mind concerning medication

We do not criticize anyone for looking for ADHD treatments that do not involve drugs, but you require to be open to the possibility that they may be necessary eventually.

Talk with your child's doctor to try and also figure out the very best Rx for them, as well as do your research study. If something does not appear right with one medication, it's your right as your child's supporter to seek out second opinions.

Many children do thrive when the appropriate combination of medications is suggested, yet these need always to be taken as a component of a broader, customized therapy strategy.

On the whole, parents raising children that have ADHD have a lot of options when it pertains to managing their child's signs and symptoms.

Coming to be an educated as well as an included parent is the first step, followed by developing an active support group through therapists, doctors, teachers, and also other caregivers.

Make sure your young person always recognizes that you're on their side, which you'll do every little thing you can to support them as they go through life with ADHD.

Also, do not forget to remember to take care of yourself. Even taking a couple of minutes to high-five yourself will make you a far better parent day in day out.

THE MYTHS AND ALSO FACTS ABOUT ADHD

Attention deficit disorder has been commonly questioned over for the last number of years as more and more children are being diagnosed. Some individuals believe that people with ADHD slouch, are stupid, and lack will power. Nonetheless, ADHD has been identified by the National Institute of Health and also the United States division of Education as a naturally based disorder. Most often, ADHD is identified in children; however, since 1978, adults have been formally diagnosed with adult ADHD too. It is evident,mainly because the majority of children who are identified with ADHD will undoubtedly mature with the very same condition. To much better understand ADHD in its entirety, you require to comprehend what is a misconception as well as what is the reality.

MYTH: ADHD is not a genuine issue. ADHD is an absence of self-control.

FACT: ADHD is a neuro-behavioral developing problem. It is a chemical imbalance in the management systems of the brain. ADHD is a legit diagnosis by significant medical, emotional, and also educational organizations utilize the Diagnostic and Statistical Manual of Mental Disorders. It is likewise recognized by the NIH as well as the United States Department of Education as a naturally based chemical discrepancy of natural chemicals in the brain.

MYTH: ADHD only influences boys.

FACT: Boys and girls are equally as most likely to be influenced by ADHD. There is nothing tried and tested that either sex is more likely to be impacted.

MYTH: Children with ADHD at some point outgrow their problem.

FACT: Approximately 70% of children detected with ADHD will remain to have signs and symptoms up through teenage years as well as 60% will continue to experience symptoms right into their adult years.

MYTH: ADHD is an outcome of bad parenting.

FACT: Parenting does not create ADHD. Children with ADHD cannot manage the impulses that make them wayward. They are not instructed to act in this manner; it is the chemistry in the brain. Some parenting methods can improve the intensity of the symptoms.

MYTH: You cannot have ADHD as an adult if you weren't identified as a child.

FACT: Some children are undiagnosed or misdiagnosed throughout the childhood years. Others can manage their symptoms as a child, consequently not ultimately experiencing or acknowledging their signs and symptoms till the adult years. The medical diagnosis of ADHD is prevalent and also ample.

MYTH: It is impossible to detect ADHD in adults precisely.

FACT: Although there isn't one test that medical diagnosis ADHD in adults, The Diagnostic, Statistical Manual of Mental Disorders and American Medical Association papers, as well as the checklist's signs and symptoms of ADHD in both children and also adults and medical professionals, have particular standards on detecting such problems.

MYTH: People with ADHD are stupid as well as careless.

FACT: Many people with ADHD have above common knowledge. The inequalities in the brain cause symptoms, which make the individual look like they are stupid or careless. Many fabulous individuals are believed to have had ADHD. Individuals who can effectively manage their condition have gone on to be CEOs as well as owners of a businesses that are still successful today.

MYTH: Everyone experiences signs of ADHD eventually; smart individuals can conquer these signs and symptoms.

FACT: ADHD has nothing to do with intelligence. Many individuals with ADHD are exceptionally highly smart. Every person can experience symptoms of ADHD. In individuals without ADHD, it's typically due to overstimulation, attitude, mood, or exhaustion. For individuals that experience ADHD, they are continuously harmed by their symptoms.

MYTH: Someone with ADHD cannot be depressed, nervous, or have psychological troubles.

FACT: Someone with ADHD is six times as most likely to experience an additional psychological or discovering condition.

MYTH: ADHD medicine drives people to abuse medications.

FACT: The prescription medicine utilized for the therapy of ADHD has been verified secure and efficient. It is more likely that neglected people with ADHD have a higher threat to misuse medicines due to habit-forming propensities. Treatment lowers the risk.

CONCLUSION

In the past, ADHD (attention-deficit/hyperactivity condition) was thought to be a problem that children had, and after that, "outgrew" before they matured. However, we now understand that ADHD is a neurological condition that spans a lifetime.

The signs and symptoms of ADHD do change with time, nonetheless. Youth hyperactivity might decrease as an adult locates healthy and balanced methods to direct their power.

Even with the shift in symptoms, ADHD can still get in the way with an adult's performance. Relationships, health, work, and funds are just a couple of locations of a person's life that might be influenced.

ADHD usually goes undiagnosed for quite some time. Numerous adults, who have felt "careless" or "scatter-brained," are surprised to discover that they have ADHD.

Whether you're a mom and dad who believes your child has ADHD, or you've just been identified with ADHD as an adult, it's essential to understand your symptoms, therapy choices, as well as the most effective techniques for living well with ADHD.

CPSIA information can be obtained
at www.ICGtesting.com
Printed in the USA
LVHW020140300421
686059LV00005B/696

9 781513 679907